Attaining Radiant Fitness

The key idea of this book is a total holism: the unity and interaction of all levels of being, m_____ nd non-material, within the individual _____ so the unity and interaction of ___ _____ at all levels with the unive_____ ____rial, energic. This unity ___ ____ ___ outer, keeping body and psy____ ___ ___ currents of life and of the natural ___ ___en as the essential secret of *youthfulness* an___ ___nce of radiant fitness.

Regardless of our physical age, so long as we are within the flow of these great currents, in our mind, our emotional-instinctual nature, and our body, we have the vital quality of youthfulness: but if we begin to close off or turn away from those contacts, in the same measure we begin to lose youthfulness. And on our abundant animation by, and oneness with, the inner and outer worlds, depends that positive quality of fitness which is the key to career success, popularity, sex appeal, fulfilled selfhood and sheer simple enjoyment of life.

Because the artificialities and the daily hassles of routine existence tend to turn our attention from the real values, *The Inner World of Fitness* leads us back by means of those natural factors in life which remain to us: air, water, sunlight, the food we eat, the world of nature, meditation, sexual love and the power of our own wishes—so that through these things we can re-link ourselves in awareness to the great non-material forces of life and of being which underlie them.

About The Author

MELITA DENNING is an internationally-recognized authority on the Western Mystery Tradition, and head of AURUM SOLIS, an organization founded in 1897 which is devoted to the study and practice of that special mystical process of psychological integration called MAGICK. She has studied Jungian psychology under the direction of a disciple of Carl Jung's friend and colleague Toni Sussmann. From 1949 through 1955 Melita traveled extensively in the Middle East, researching into the medieval order of the Knights Templar: for her historical work in this regard she was, in 1968, created Dame d'Honneur by the Swiss head of the Sovereign Military Order of the Temple of Jerusalem. She is co-author of *The Magical Philosophy*, a definitive five volume work on Western esotericism, and of *The Llewellyn Practical Guide Series*. She is listed in a number of biographical reference works, including *Who's Who in the World* and *Dictionary of International Biography*.

To Write to the Author

We cannot guarantee that every letter written to the author can be answered, but all will be forwarded to her. Both the author and the publisher appreciate hearing from readers, learning of your enjoyment and benefit from this book. Llewellyn also publishes a bi-monthly news magazine with news and reviews of practical esoteric studies and articles helpful to the student, and some readers' questions and comments to the author may be answered through this magazine's columns if permission to do is included in the original letter. The author sometimes participates in seminars and workshops, and dates and places are announced in *The Llewellyn New Times*. To write to the author, or to ask a question, write to:

Melita Denning
c/o THE LLEWELLYN NEW TIMES
P.O. Box 64383-165, St. Paul, MN 55164-0383, U.S.A.
Please enclose a self-addressed, stamped envelope for reply, or $1.00 to cover costs.

ABOUT LLEWELLYN'S NEW AGE SERIES

The "New Age"—it's a phrase we use, but what does it mean? Does it mean the changing of the Zodiacal Tides, that we are entering the Aquarian Age? Does it mean that a new Messiah is coming to correct all that is wrong and make Earth into a Garden? Probably not—but the idea of a *major change* is there, combined with awareness that Earth *can* be a Garden; that war, crime, poverty, disease, etc., are not necessary "evils".

Optimists, dreamers, scientists . . . nearly all of us believe in a "better tomorrow", and that somehow we can do things now that will make for a better future life for ourselves and for coming generations.

In one sense, we all know "there's nothing new under the Heavens", and in another sense that "every day makes a new world". The difference is in our consciousness. And this is what the New Age is all about: it's a major change in consciousness found within each of us as we learn to bring forth and manifest "powers" that Humanity has always potentially had.

Evolution moves in "leaps". Individuals struggle to develop talents and powers, and their efforts build a "power bank" in the Collective Unconsciousness, the "soul" of Humanity that suddenly makes these same talents and powers easier access for the majority.

Those who talk about a New Age believe a new level of consciousness is becoming accessible that will allow anyone to manifest powers previously restricted to the few who had worked strenuously for them: powers such as Healing (for self and others), Creative Visualization, Psychic Perception, Out-of-Body Consciousness and more.

You still have to learn the 'rules' for developing and applying these powers, but it is more like a "relearning" than a *new* learning, because with the New Age it is as if the basis for these had become genetic.

The books in the New Age series are as much about ATTITUDE and AWARENESS as they are about the "mechanics" for learning and using Psychic, Mental, Spiritual, or Parapsychological Powers. Understanding that the Human Being is indeed a "potential god" is the first step towards the realization of that potential: expressing in outer life the inner creative powers.

Other Books From Melita Denning, Co-Authored with Osborne Phillips

The Magical Philosophy*—A Study of the Western Mystery Tradition
    Book I, *Robe and Ring*, 1974
    Book II, *The Apparel of High Magick*, 1975
    Book III, *The Sword and the Serpent*, 1975
    Book IV, *The Triumph of Light*, 1978
    Book V, *Mysteria Magica*, 1982

The Llewellyn Practical Guide(s) to:
    Astral Projection, 1979
    Creative Visualization, 1980
    Psychic Self-Defense & Well-Being, 1980
    The Development of Psychic Powers, 1981
    The Magick of Sex, 1982
    The Magick of the Tarot, 1983

The Llewellyn Mystery Religion Series:
    Voudoun Fire: The Living Reality of Mystical Religion

The Llewellyn Deep Mind Tape(s) for:
    Astral Projection and the Out-of-Body Experience, 1981

The Llewellyn Inner Guide(s) to:
    Magical States of Consciousness, 1985

The Llewellyn Inner Guide Tape(s):
    Paths to Inner Worlds, Series I (tapes—Paths 32 to 24), 1985

Other Books and Tapes Forthcoming:
    The Llewellyn Inner Guide to Planetary Magick
    The Llewellyn Practical Guide to Talismanic Magick
    The Magical Philosophy, Revised, in Three Volumes
    Fire Out of Eden
    Evocation of the Gods
    Moving with Power
    The World of Celtic Magic
    The Inner World of Fitness (by Melita Denning)

Also forthcoming:
    A Correspondence Course in the Western Esoteric Tradition

Llewellyn's New Age Series

The Inner World of Fitness

Melita Denning

1987
Llewellyn Publications
St. Paul, Minnesota, 55164-0384, U.S.A.

International Standard Book Number: 0-87542-165-2
Library of Congress Catalog Number: 85-45281

First Edition, 1986
First Printing, 1986
Second Printing, 1987

Library of Congress Cataloging-in-Publication Data
Denning, Melita.
    The inner world of fitness.

    (Llewellyn's new age series)
    1. Health.   2. Holistic medicine.   3. Psychical research.   4.
Physical fitness.   I. Title.   II. Series.
RA776.5.D45   1986   613.8   85-45281
ISBN 0-87542-165-2

Cover Design: Terry Buske and Animation Services
Illustrations: Leslie Rogalski

Produced by Llewellyn Publications
Typography and Art property of Chester-Kent, Inc.

Published by
LLEWELLYN PUBLICATIONS
A Division of Chester-Kent, Inc.
P.O. Box 64383
St. Paul, MN 55164-0383, U.S.A.

Printed in the United States of America

TABLE OF CONTENTS

Chapter 5: Come With Bows Bent . . .

a special mirror for this practice. Your Deep Mind speaks in your dreams. The full-length mirror: its help in your exercise schedule. Finally: Radiant Fitness and Radiant Fun.

Appendix A   On Fasting
The fashion in fasting. Good and bad reasons for fasting. Effective fasting: what you can gain from it. Two ways to fast effectively. Choosing the right time for your fast.

Appendix B   The Tropical Banana Breakfast
An elusive legend. The words of one who knew. What the Breakfast is and why it works. Practical hints and some delicious variations.

Appendix C   A Calm Look at AIDS
History's roll-call of killer maladies. The clouds of unreason. Keep abreast of known facts! AIDS, a virus. The positive protective powers of good health, fitness, optimism.

Chapter One

THERE IS ONE LESSON . . .

There is one lesson at all Times and Places —
One changeless Truth on all things changing writ,
For boys and girls, men, women, nations, races —
Be fit — be fit! And, once again, be fit!
Rudyard Kipling, "A Preface"

Fitness, in itself, is a magical word these days, and this is no surprise. Think of energy, happiness, the sparkle of a mind and body acting in harmony, and you think of fitness. Think of the grace of strong but relaxed movement, the poise, optimism and good humor which radiate from the possessor of inner well-being and self-assurance, and again you think of fitness. Fitness is all these things besides bright eyes, a clear skin and a swinging step.

Fitness is, by the very positive nature of the word, something over and above "health". To be "healthy" is to be whole, *healed:* to be without malady. To be "fit" is to be ready, able to cope — fit for action, fit for life! Fitness is health in abundance, life in abundance: and that, in truth, is what all life desires.

Unconquerable Youth

The idea of fitness is inseparable from the idea of *youth*,

1

of young adulthood. Granted, we all know people whose birth certificates show them to be far from "young", yet whose fitness is vibrant. But these very people are living illustrations of the point. No matter what the documentation says, no matter what color their hair may be or how much the laughter lines at the corners of eyes and mouth may have deepened, these people move in an aura of unconquerable youth: nobody who knows them thinks at all of their physical age. More, they have youth without the fears and uncertainties with which physical youth is so often troubled. By reason of their fitness and their long experience in meeting life's challenges they have found themselves, and have seen more deeply within than to need reassurance from outward sources.

To Inspire Confidence

The fit person not only benefits directly from the vitality, zest and joy which fitness brings: there are also indirect, but very real and important, "bonus" benefits which arise from the attitude of other people. The fit person inspires confidence, attracts liking and friendship. He or she impresses others as being capable, reliable and fair minded.

This impression, although usually wholly emotional and perhaps not even consciously received, yet makes good sense, too. One who so evidently knows how to live his or her own life to good advantage is, at the least, one who has no likely motive to injure others and, at best, a person to be regarded as a tower of strength and of good counsel.

At the same time, any beholders who may themselves be seeking for a potential victim, whether for trickery or even for violence, are likely to be put off when they become aware of the fit person's assurance and inner power.

The Protective Power of Fitness

Here, too, the reason is simple. Human predators and

parasites, like any other predators and parasites, are not seeking adventure or trying to make trouble for them selves. They want the easiest pickings. The visible confidence of the fit person is, itself, a deterrent, and psychically, the well-developed defensive aura is a real shield against predatory imaginings. (At the same time, no matter how great your self-confidence, you are not advised to *swagger*. The man or woman who makes too crude a display of strength may arouse the resentment of a bold assailant, or may tempt a more cunning enemy to reflect that bravado sometimes masks hidden weakness. Let your confidence radiate *naturally*.)*

Fitness and Attractiveness

The positive "bonus" benefits of radiant fitness are many. Are you looking for a lover? *Fitness attracts.* Your fitness proclaims you are a good person to be with, a fun person, not preoccupied with any inner woes. "Hearts that are happy are loving and kind," says the old song — and fitness is a large ingredient in happiness.

Besides, if you radiate fitness, you will not only attract. Chances are you'll attract the right kind of partner. The fit young woman is not likely to attract the chauvinist who is seeking an "old fashioned" girl he can impress and dominate — in fact she'll probably scare him off! The fit young man is not likely to attract the over-maternal, basically selfish sort of woman who'll want to run his career and his whole life for him.

Certainly, seeking the right partner has a variety of pitfalls both for men and for women, but there we see two frequent bogies promptly dealt with. The cultivation of fitness brings together women and men who can regard each other with mutual respect, who can look for a true sharing

---

*The subject of the protective aura, with a range of practices for its development and activation, is explained in detail in *The Llewellyn Practical Guide to Psychic Self-Defense and Well-Being*. That book, like the present one, is a self-contained manual on its own subject area, but the two can be used together very effectively.

of activities and interests, who can hope to build together a genuine partnership in life.

Fitness and the Employment Scene

In the business world, fitness wins more and bigger prizes than are generally credited to its influence. The manager, or executive, who seems to bring an electric current or a breath of fresh air into office or board room wields an instantaneous impact and power about which no more need be said. But at other levels too, *fitness is strength.*

People who hire staff, people concerned in promoting staff, appreciate fitness. Some reasons for this are simple and obvious. A fit person will not take too many days' sick leave. A fit person will have the energy and application to make a good thing of his or her job. Even for those plain reasons, the glow of radiant fitness is a valuable asset to have; after all, everyone who is competing for a particular job, or a particular promotion, is likely to take care to project an image of normal good health. Radiant fitness commends itself more positively, as well as on a broader basis.

Management may or may not consciously know something about the group aura which develops around, emanates from, every group of persons who regularly work or play together. These days, management people likely know many more things than show up in the qualifications they exhibit. But even if they have never heard of the group aura by name, they know from experience that any one group of people (office, class, baseball team, choir or what have you) develops a definite overall "spirit" which is not quite like that of any other similar group, and that this "spirit" may be one which benefits the joint effort and the individual members or it may be the reverse. And not only does this invisible factor influence to some extent each individual member, but each individual member likewise contributes something to it.

To "it" — that is, to the group aura — the radiantly fit member of the staff, no matter what his or her official function in the organization, will contribute positive and potent qualities, likely to enhance the motivation and performance of the whole group. Employers are for the most part acutely aware of the benefits of taking on, or of promoting, such a person.

Fitness and P.R.

Supposing in your work you need to meet members of the public: as a technician perhaps, or as a salesperson. With increased vitality, energy, fitness, you can certainly do more and better work. But, again, that is not all!

With radiant fitness, you will inspire greater confidence. People will pay more attention to what you say and do. People will *enjoy* watching you work, listening to what you tell them. And in sales, or in the demonstration of equipment, these are matters of paramount importance. These factors will influence people's decision to buy. They will influence, time after time — *and quite justly* — the general opinion as to the thoroughness of your demonstrations, the clarity of your explanations and instructions.

That is only reasonable. For if you had spoken exactly the same words in a flat, weary voice, or performed exactly the same actions in a listless manner; above all, if the vitality and dynamism of your personality had not held them, most people would hardly be certain of what you said or did, still less would they feel sufficient interest to ask questions.

The same power of holding attention is equally important if your work involves counseling for instance, or coaching, or teaching school. Children and adults alike respond to fitness.

Radiant Fitness for the Handicapped

For anyone physically handicapped in any measure,

the extra boost to morale and to the projected self-image which can be gained with fitness is likely to be of great and special value. The problem here, remarkably enough, is not often at its most acute for people with serious disabilities. Partly as a result of skilled help in rehabilitation, partly through the natural response of body and psyche to a massive emergency situation, it happens that amputees, victims of paralysis, and the blind (to take a few examples) often show great resources of both body and psyche, great morale, and do much to cheer and hearten others besides themselves.

The people who are frequently the most hurt, sometimes almost psychically disabled by their personal experiences, are some with relatively minor handicaps. Such troubles can in some cases wreck a person's self-image without calling forth, either in the sufferers personally or in friends and neighbors, any clear-cut conviction of having a nameable trouble to deal with. The person whose powers of vision, while adequate for many purposes, are impaired in a way which would put a driver's license out of the question, could be an example here; another could be the would-be athlete, perhaps a person of great strength and stamina, whose genes came up with a pattern of short legs and long torso instead of the preferred alternative. Often people find themselves disqualified, by maybe only a single physical factor which nevertheless they are powerless to change, from a career or an avocation otherwise ideally suitable for them.

To all who feel that through some disability their self-image, or their power of self-expression through physical life, has been impaired, the development of fitness, and self-manifestation through fitness, is seriously commended. It is not offered as a kind of "consolation prize", for it is not offered to these distressed people alone. In this book it is proposed to set forth — for the use of any and every person who is by ordinary standards in a state of good health — a plan of traditional means for the enhancement and maintenance of fitness, and, since the basis of fitness belong to the psyche as well as to the body, this plan is to aid in bringing body and psyche into closer harmony to provide a better, more vital, combined instrument of expression for the person.

Everybody Smile!

So this is for the person who is looking forward to a rimwalk at Grand Canyon, and for the person who failed an important medical because of something constitutional. It is for the person in a wheelchair, and the person who is "tied" to a desk for longer hours than are good for anyone. It is for the prospective next Miss (or Mr.) Cosmos, and also for anyone who has just gathered that the ballet class has no enthusiasm about his or her continued attendance. And — to keep to one sex for the moment because the other really has no equivalent — it is for the housewife and mother who wants, between chores, to revitalize herself in time for next Thanksgiving/Christmas/swimsuit season.

It is likewise for the person who has no special objective or problem, but who enjoys living and is interested in doing just that as thoroughly and systematically as possible.

Fitness and Sickness

Obviously, if you have any real sickness your doctor is the right authority to consult. Equally obviously, if 'flu or some other virus or bug gets you down, you will not for the time being feel particularly "radiant", except perhaps in the manner of the luminous Rudolph. But your fitness program should certainly help you throw off such maladies more quickly than you otherwise would; and, other things being equal, it ought also to reduce the frequency of winter colds, etc. — unless you hardly ever get them anyway!

Simplifying the Data

The link between mind and body in matters of health and physical performance is being generally admitted nowadays. Much research is being done, and statistics are being produced, to show how the mind influences the body to produce healing, for instance, in a wide range of different cases, and how in various sports and athletic practices the action of the body in turn produces altered states of consciousness. (To call these altered states a "high", as is sometimes done, would seem to be a misnomer unless it is claimed that in such cases the exercitant gets "high" on adrenalin, oxygen or other factor in the bloodstream. But altered states there must be, if the exercise is sufficient, as a result of the prolongation of attention thereto. The long distance runner, for instance, is as effectively encapsuled in the action as is a person in a "rebirthing" tank.)

The whole matter of the mind-body exchange, interesting though the researches are, is at once much simplified if we start from the fact that in every inquiry of this kind we are dealing with a living person, a psycho-physical unit in which a continual cause-and-effect exchange — emotion, instinct, gland, nerve, instinct, emotion again — goes on throughout life, waking or sleeping, perceived or unperceived. For our present purpose — an examination of fitness — one of the most notable facts which present-day researches are confirming over and over, is that bodily action of all sorts is directly controlled and regulated by the sympathetic nerves and the unconscious levels of the mind.

Try This Yourself

When the conscious mind has an intention of directing the body in any way, it must establish contact with those levels of the psycho-physical unit which are outside its direct dominion, and must work through them. This takes practice. Mostly we establish, early in life, the contacts necessary to govern those actions which are most important to us, and thereafter forget the learning process and cherish the illusion that in some matters at least the conscious mind governs the body directly.

You can test this illusion quite simply. Take a piece of paper and write your name on it — just "your usual signature" as the banks say. Your signature is thoroughly familiar to you, your mind wills your hand to write it, and there it is on paper.

Now just transfer the pen to your other hand and repeat the process. Unless you have always been ambidextrous, or unless you've taken trouble to train your weaker hand in certain skills to be prepared for possible emergencies, no matter how mature and capable a person you are, the second signature is likely to look like a child's early efforts. Why? The hand is there, the will and intellect are there to direct it. But the hand is not responding adequately, because the message and the "know-how" communicated by the conscious mind are not fully getting through to it. The connecting link has not been cultivated.

Health is Wholeness

The tendency of many people, in keeping up with the pace of daily life, is to "cut themselves in half" leaving the unconscious functions of the personality to run one set of activities while the conscious functions run a different set. It might be hoped that in this way each section might do its own work more successfully, but in fact this is not the result. The result is a medley of absentmindedness, unfocused anxiety, "floating guilt" (which is mostly the same thing as the anxiety), stress, bad digestion and problems of circulation, lungs and heart. This is no paradox; the personality, or the person, is designed to operate as a unity. To glance at a positive aspect of the picture: when we set out to teach a person how, deliberately, to separate the consciousness from the body in Astral Projection, the early training is devoted to ensuring that through various practices the student is enabled to energize himself or herself effectively at all levels, as a unity. Nor does the act of projection sunder that unity; it is not the "astral body" as a whole, but only a "vehicle" of astral substance, in which the consciousness makes its expedition out-of-the-body.

While on the topic of astral projection, it may be mentioned that in all the instances which have come to our knowledge of spontaneous projection as a result of sickness, of anesthesia or of sudden accident, the evidence has been of a well-organized constitution and a strong body-psyche bond. Even a seemingly fragile person can have great stamina in this way, though most of the people we have known about have been markedly robust.

That woman was no weakling who, thrown from her horse during a cross-country race, was astonished to see her unconscious body lying upon the ground before her. Nor was the soldier who, stricken with fever in the Far Eastern jungles, yet stumbled along with the rest of his party. Repeatedly, while the fever was with him, he saw an unknown "extra man" — whose face he never glimpsed — moving just ahead of him; only some years later, as a veteran, he once more caught sight of that back in a tailor's mirror and realized it was his own.

The many similar instances of "autoscopy" (seeing one's own body) which are revealed in recent investigations of the "Near Death Experience" — recounted, necessarily, by survivors — tend to the same conclusion. Projection of consciousness does not show any weakness of the relationship between body and psyche.

Conscious and Unconscious

We are not, then, considering body and psyche as being by nature sharply divided: indeed, in nature two adjacent phenomena hardly ever are sharply divided. There is another distinction, however, which is important for us: "conscious" and "unconscious". Some functions of the psyche are conscious. Always, as the little handwriting test above illustrates, it is the unconscious functions which are vital to communication between the different levels of our being.

These unconscious functions, therefore, have great importance to us in this matter of fitness, for here we must communicate our conscious will to the other levels of our being, so that no injurious barriers may exist between level and level.

The Secret of Youth

In youth, there are no such barriers. Candid thought and vivid emotion, pulse of instinct, wing of spirit and the joy that sings in blood and sinew: youth is all these together, rejecting none. The older person who keeps youthfulness may be wiser and more discerning than youth itself, may be more humorous too, but still there too, we see the same directness, the same spontaneity. The closing of doors in the soul, irrespective of a person's age, is in some measure youth's fading. This may come through fear or through bitterness, but often it comes simply through incomprehension of the true values involved, and a belief that every moment can be given to outward things without any harm resulting. Health may survive in its essentials but fitness goes; for fitness involves energy in movement, energy flowing through body and psyche unhindered. Fitness — radiant fitness — is the product of "aliveness" coursing through all the levels of being.

To show you how to keep, enhance or regain this

radiant and vibrant quality of life is the purpose of this book.

Now we come to the Magick

If you could communicate easily with all the levels of your being, you could have perfect fitness for the commanding, but as we have seen, this is seldom the case. You have to work through your unconscious faculties, through your Deep Mind, and your Deep Mind being by the nature of things irrational, if you sit down and address it in rational terms alone you are not likely to have much success. Nor is hypnosis — even self-hypnosis — likely to be a very satisfactory method, if it is used, as is sometimes the case, to "convince" the Deep Mind that it wants something which really it doesn't want, or vice versa.

A child was once taken to the store for a pair of shoes, and she set her heart on a patent-leather pair with big square buckles on the instep. Her mother told her she didn't really want those, they weren't "sensible" and the child could see no flaw in her mother's reasoning, so the "sensible" shoes were bought instead. But that night, after being put to bed and sleeping for perhaps an hour, the child woke up and proceeded to cry inconsolably for the buckle-shoes. The mother renewed her reasonable arguments, but, this time, was answered only by an inflexible "I want them!" So, in the morning, the "sensible" shoes had to be taken back, and the exchange made.

That is frequently what happens when by means of hypnosis or other coercion the unconscious mind is led to make a false denial of its desires and inclinations. All will seem to be well until the reaction sets in, but, when it does, that which Reason wanted to alter will be found more firmly entrenched than ever, and means will be hard to find that will shift it.

Even in the simplest things there is but one way to

"speak" to your Deep Mind effectively, and that is by means of symbolism (visible, imagined or enacted) and of the desirable reward, the incentive. Certainly you can use words — aloud, if you like — either in a period of quiet, simple meditation or in the course of performing a magical technique you may know. These things help, chiefly by helping you give a fine focal point to your will and intention; but the method given in this present book is equally potent and effective, while making more use of symbolism.

The Potent Language of Symbol

There are symbols which are so powerfully linked to what they symbolize that if you mean them so (and sometimes even if you know nothing about it) they *produce* the effects which they *represent*. To put it in a more sophisticated way, they show forth a "language" which your Deep Mind intrinsically understands, and your Deep Mind — the limits of whose power nobody has as yet been able to gauge — will achieve, or will open itself to receive, that which is symbolized. Tremendous magical use can be made of these symbols. The Church uses some of them — water for cleansing, bread to nourish and so on — and some of them have been used in innumerable religions: wine to outpass rationality, fire for transformation and transition. But the world in which we live is full of such symbols, and the comprehension and acceptance of them, deeper than consciousness, is a part of our life.

In this book you will be shown how to use a number of these symbols to win the co-operation of your Deep Mind to empower your work for fitness. The symbols, like the bread and the fire and so on, are good things in themselves, but the magical empowerment they will bring to you is even better.

In the Canary Islands before the Spaniards changed

the religion, the native people had a very simple and strong religion of their own. It was based on the unity of all life, the unity of all that is: consequently, when these people performed a ceremony, they did not always say in words what more than the physical action was implied. The non-material side could be understood to follow spontaneously by virtue of the unity of the people with the All.

For instance, a *Magada* — a priestess — would pour water over the head of a new-born child, solemnly saying something like "Wash in water, and be you clean!"

Even thus, in the practices which follow in this book, sometimes there will be words to state precisely the deeper purposes underlying the obvious physical purpose, and sometimes there will not. If there are not, you can add them if you like, but this is not always an advantage, for you may be limiting to one interpretation a symbol which, of itself, can function in many ways and at different levels. So — unless you have your own reason to direct a practice to a very specific purpose — reflect carefully upon the matter before adding words.

Unity of All Life

You have here, then, powerful magical means as well as physical ones for re-linking the levels of your own being for radiant fitness. But that is not all the help you have.

You are not, in any case, an isolated unit. Through your Higher Self you are linked, however unconsciously it may be, to the glorious and infinite World of the Divine. You are surrounded — again, it may be, unconsciously — by a vast number of unseen helpers and well wishers, Elder Sisters and Brothers both human and other. You are one with the human race, and one with the life of this planet, and one with all the forces of the cosmos which work in you and through you.

When you free yourself from the inner barriers and let

the life forces within you flow and circulate as they should, you are also granting more liberal ways to the flow and circulation through your being of the life forces and powers of the larger universe of which you are a part. This, with time and practice, can bring you to a greater conscious awareness of them, a joyful comprehension of their harmony and, where need be, a self-adjustment accordingly. This cosmic expansion of selfhood is a part of our rightful heritage, and is, in fact, the logical ultimate development of the concept of Fitness. We are from the beginning a part of the All, but our acceptance and realization of it must be through our own will.

Chapter Two

LO, THE MOST EXCELLENT SUN

> Lo, the most excellent sun so calm and haughty,
> The violet and purple morn with just-felt breezes,
> The gentle soft-born measureless light,
> The miracle spreading bathing all, the fulfilled noon . . .
> *Walt Whitman, "When lilacs last"*

What is the most wonderful thing in the world? Each person, according to individual interests and temperament, in pondering that question, might come up with a whole list of astonishing things, mysterious things, beautiful things, and there would be a great variety of lists. Yet, in any such list, surely *Light* would merit a high place; perhaps the highest place among phenomena which are actually within our experience.

Light is, essentially, a manifestation of energy, of visible radiant energy. Not only is the presence of light necessary for the sense of sight to function, it is by the stimulating effect of light that the very faculty of sight has come into being.

Light and Love

The importance of *looking* is basic to life's great experi-

17

ences. We look, and wonder; we look, and learn; we look, and love. Centuries of love songs have been written on the theme of lovers gazing into each other's eyes, but that is not the only kind of love to be thus nourished. According to our present day researchers, in the "bonding" of mother and child — the process by which a biological relationship becomes a true commitment of the will on either side — a major part is played by "eye contact", the exchange of gaze. It is noteworthy that the researchers use the word "contact" here. Touch is the supreme thing. For blind people, or in the dark, the sense of touch not only fulfils its own purposes but also takes the place of sight; for sighted folk in the light, sight is a form of touch, of contact. The old philosophers of love were not far wrong when they described physical beams of light traveling from the eyes of one lover to enter into the eyes of the other.

If sight is so important in these two vital forms of love, we can infer an equal importance for it in other relationships. Indeed, everyday speech suggests this is so. If you are going to visit or meet a friend, you may be planning a long conversation, maybe a meal or a few drinks together, some kind of shared activity, but quite often you say of it, "I am going to see So-and-so." If you are going to "see" someone in hospital, where really no form of shared activity is possible except to help eat the grapes, the literal sense of the word is revealed with particular force. You go to look, to satisfy yourself as to the invalid's progress, and also to hearten her or him with your presence, and often the sick person will remark on the joy of *seeing* you.

For all this we are indebted, directly and indirectly, to light. But our debt is greater even than that. Much scientific inquiry and speculation is directed to the origins of life itself; specifically, the origins of the particular mode of life existing as a biological phenomenon on this planet.* These speculations are of great interest, for the concept of life as a divine and spiritual reality is in no way opposed to that of an animate earthly "vehicle" evolving perilously upwards to meet it.

Light and Life

Certainly there was a time when life was not present upon this planet. Then, beginning with very simple and unevolved forms, life begins to be manifest. How did the all-important change come about? The mineral world existing before the appearance of life was the arena of mighty forces: great electrical storms, and powerful radioactivity in metals and other substances which are now found only in an inert, exhausted form. A passage in *The Magical Philosophy* tells the story:

"For how many ages this stage of development continues we cannot say, but amino acids and other nitrogen compounds are the foundation of protein, and protein molecules are the foundation of life, to which the other chemicals are also necessary. The Sun . . . rays down its warm and vital light upon the seas. There the amino acids and the other minerals react and conjugate, bound up with the hydrocarbon colloids. The tensions in colloidal droplets, the inherent molecular rhythms of crystalline substances, provide recurring lines of force in radial and segmented quasi-organic forms: long before life is present, the patterns in which life is maintained are established. And then at last, almost imperceptibly, the new factor is produced: life has come into being. From the colloidal droplet, the single-celled organism evolves in the protozoic slime."†

---

*It is not intended to imply that biological life exists nowhere in the Cosmos but on this planet. There is no evidence either way. For different atmospheres, pressures and degrees of light, the chemistry would need to be different from ours, but we have no reason to suppose ours is the only viable system. Before science can speculate on the nature of such xenobic forms however, it would need first to find them and to identify them *by test methods which would not in any case instantly destroy them.* "There's the rub."

†From *The Sword and the Serpent* (Book III of *The Magical Philosophy*) Chapter II, "Genesis 1:1-20 revised."

Inevitably it is the light and heat, the energy of the Sun, which is the critical and decisive factor among all the factors involved in this matter. There is the less inclination to hesitate regarding this hypothesis, because we see that in every other respect, no matter how far we may have evolved, our earthly lives remain entirely dependent upon the Sun.

Life amid Eternal Snows

Nowhere is this dependence more dramatically demonstrated than in arctic and antarctic regions. With the seasonal tilt of the respective poles towards or away from the sun, the temperature in both regions varies through the year over an extraordinarily wide range, and life of all kinds flourishes tropically or practically vanishes accordingly. The inner heat of the earth is, from the evidence, certainly not enough in itself to sustain any of the more evolved life-forms, except in a few places where volcanic activity produces hot springs. That type of ecology, however, is of extremely limited range.

There is a species of small fish, for instance, whose only habitat in the world consists of a few yards in a particular Antarctic river; the limited few yards in which the water is neither too hot nor too cold for their survival. And even those fish are dependent upon sunlight for the development of the organisms on which they feed.

Eating and Drinking Sunlight

Consider your own diet. The question is not, at this time, what or how you would do well to eat and drink, that is to come in Chapter 7. All you are asked to review at the moment is what in fact you do eat and drink and where it comes from. Whether you eat green vegetables, root vegetables, cereals (with which such things as bread and pasta can be included), nuts, meat, dairy products or fruit, you get back to your dependence on the action of sunlight in one move or two at most. Admittedly, unless you grow your own salad vegetables, the probability now is that the first daylight to shine on the ones you have was when they were brought out for shipping to the stores, but the whole race of lettuces, celery, tomatoes and what have you, needed to grow in sunlight for ages to get as far as this sophisticated century, and even the ones you eat have required for their growth a decent commercial imitation of sunlight. And, of course, you are presumably not trying to live on salad vegetables.

If you drink anything but plain water, you are at once indebted to the sunlight whether you swallow milk, coffee, tea, wine, beer, spirits, or fruit or vegetable juices. Even those very synthetic "soft drinks" whose highest virtues seem generally to be expressed as negatives are likely to contain at least a percentage of lemon or sugar, and/or some other product of the vegetable kingdom.

Breathing Sunlight

So you live by sunlight, you eat and drink sunlight. (And incidentally, if your clothing contains any natural fabric, or even some synthetics such as rayon, you owe that to the sunlight too, directly or at a simple remove.) Furthermore — and this is particularly important to reflect upon — *you breathe sunlight.*

Sunlight is antiseptic. It can break down many substances, chiefly by means of its ultraviolet component, which is one reason why lotions and similar preparations which are meant to be kept, are usually supplied in a colored bottle or jar and should be kept in a cool dark place. But sometimes this destructive quality is a good thing, and sunlight shining through the air does a great deal to destroy, or at least to put out of action, many of the harmful bacteria, mold and fungal spores which float in the atmosphere.

Rain helps to purify the air. Trees and other green plants help replenish the air with the oxygen they exhale. Somewhat further on in this book, in Chapter 4, there will be more about Air and its natural and magical functions in relation to fitness. Just now, however, the thing to reflect upon is Air as carrying the warm, strong, purifying and vitalizing power of sunlight.

Imagine . . .

Picture that you are out of doors, in open, grassy land, with a few trees here and there. You stand on the top of a gentle grassy hill, the sky is blue, clear but not very intense in color. There is very little breeze, and the sun shines down from directly overhead so that the air is filled with pale golden light; warm, vibrant, life-giving. You welcome it, you take a slow, deep breath of it, opening your whole being to the sunlight and absorbing it into yourself. You feel the sunlight almost tingling in your veins, spreading a deep sense of well-being; you see it as it glows in your heart, and you feel the happiness and contentment it brings.

This imagination may come very easily to you, whether because you have had practice in such meditations, or because you are something of an outdoorsperson. If it does not come easily, you should work at it, either by repeatedly imagining it, or, if possible, by going outdoors and doing the thing itself in the most suitable surroundings you can find. However practiced you are in more "abstract" forms of meditation, it is good, whenever the circumstances are right, to renew the experience of this kind of natural reality.

Magical Creativity

Magick can be worked in many different ways, some of them far removed from ordinary life. But, especially when you want the results of your magick to be manifest at the earthly level (as you certainly do with fitness), it's good to keep it "earthed" at various points: linked to natural experience in some way. You need not only to make your action real, you want every part of you to be able to share in knowing, feeling, living its reality. In doing this, your greatest helper is your imagination, so you should keep your imagination well nourished. Breathing in sunlight, filling yourself with it, is an excellent magical reality to begin on.

Modifications of Light

Before we go on to build further on that foundation, there is more to say about light. We need to consider the moon, the planets and the stars.

The light we receive from the moon and the planets is, as we know, reflected from the sun. That, however, does not mean it is simply sunlight. Each planet receives the light of the sun from a different distance in space, due to the different orbits of those planets. Each planet has a different convexity of surface, and a different type of surface. In what way such factors as these affect the light which is reflected to us from the planets we cannot readily say, but it is not surprising that the light is in each instance considerably modified. Nor, considered in this way, is it really surprising that each of these modified lights affects us in a different way, just as the vibrations of different musical notes, or of different colors, affect us differently.

One of the chief divergences between science and magick is that magick can work with effects, not necessarily understanding all the causes. Sometimes the causes come eventually to be known, and then what was magick passes into the domain of science. But, unfortunately, that isn't all that happens, because when the intellect takes over the imagination tends to stand back, and so the scientific work is usually done by part of a person whereas the magick was done by a whole person. However, it is beginning to be admitted now that different sounds have their specific effects on people, and that so do different colors. And, for that matter, it is beginning to be perceived that there is reality to the different planetary influences.

So sunlight reflected to us by some other body in our solar system is no longer just sunlight. In fact, the analogy with color is worth pursuing a little further, because color also is a modification of light. If you pass white light through a prism, it is split into the seven colors of the spectrum. Each of those colors is, certainly, a part of white light. But nonetheless, each of those colors will produce its own special emotional and subtle physical effects on whoever may be immersed in that color alone, so that its origin as a component of white light becomes practically irrelevant. We can consider the planetary modifications of sunlight in a somewhat similar manner.

With regard to the moon, which is so much nearer to Earth than any of the planets, some definite statements can be made at once. We can put a name to at least one important difference between moonlight and the sunlight which the moon receives: moonlight is *polarized*. That is to say, the moon's light — or a proportion of it — comes at you like a volley of arrows. One cause of this is the moon's closeness to us, and one of its main effects is that we, and indeed all living things on Earth, are affected by the moon's rays to a much greater extent than its relatively weak light would seem to warrant.

This Experiment is Optional

If you want a more distinct understanding of this action of moonlight, walk close by a lawn sprinkler in operation. (To get the full effect of this, you really need to do it absentmindedly, not noticing until you are hit.) What it feels like is a battery of water pistols, charged with just-melted ice, all deliberately and with malice aimed straight at you. Supposing, however, you were to pass the same sprink-ler at a distance of about eight feet, say, when the water-drops have had a chance to fan out and to be affected by other forces, such as gravity and maybe a breeze, you would realize there's nothing violent or intense about it, and certainly no personal aggression. The water is losing its polarization.

The Domain of the Moon

The moon can, of course, do beautiful things for you, but they are mostly very much below the level of conscious-ness. Think of the successes of gardeners who work accord-ing to the phases and zodiacal signs of the moon; this is no "old wives' tale" but has been demonstrated over and over. Think not only of the magically powerful light of the moon, but of the lunar magnetism which sways the tides. At the physical level, at the vegetative level of life, at the instinc-tual level below the threshold of consciousness, and in the Astral World of dreams and visions, wishes and fantasies, that is where the moon works for you, in her own domain.

You can work with her for your own benefit, and work closely with her if you know the secrets of "what" and "when". To study this for a specific objective, such as fit-ness, can be very rewarding, for in this much of your con-cern is with those physical and instinctual levels which it is so hard to reach consciously. To do this a simple guide, such as Llewellyn's *Moon Sign Book,* will give what you need. But if, at first, you want to work on simpler lines than those, then remember this rule. When you have occasion to invoke or employ the lunar powers in any way, it's best to avoid doing so when the moon is waning.

Everyone agrees that to work for something you want, or something you have but wish to increase, or for some-thing particularly associated with the moon, the right time is the "first half" of the Moon, from the New Moon up to the

Full. About the time that follows the Full Moon, however, opinions differ. Some people say, use that time to deal with things you want to get rid of, like corns or smoking. We'd say, do those things on the Full Moon, or use the positive power of another luminary instead. The time of the moon's waning might work out, or it might not. You are then using a weak, uncertain and unreliable force, like having your hair cut with blunt instruments. (They are not "malefic", any more than the waning moon is, but the results can be unsatisfactory.)

Planets and Zodiac

The planetary powers — the cosmic powers themselves which are represented by the traditional "Seven Planets" (which include sun and moon)* have their archetypal counterparts deep within the psyche. It is through these counterparts that the planetary powers influence us, a fact which has been realized by the more profound astrologers for centuries. (Indeed, any external spiritual force which in any way influences us, whether to our good or harm, can only do so by means of some counterpart, or image, established within our psyche — inside our defenses, so to speak — either naturally as with the planetary and zodiacal forces, or by stimulating our imagination to create such an image).

Our bodies, however, are governed by the astral level of our psyche, and our "astral body", being a part of the astral world just as our physical body is a part of the material world, is strongly affected — as is the whole astral world —by the zodiacal influences, those twelve powerful and distinctive currents of force which are differently awakened and activated according both to their own nature and

---

*The "new planets", i.e., those discovered in recent times, are astrologically regarded as "higher octaves" of certain of the traditional ones, with which they share rulership of the relevant zodiacal signs. They therefore do not affect the traditional plan, but their co-rulership is shown on the ensuing table as it may be of high significance in some instances.

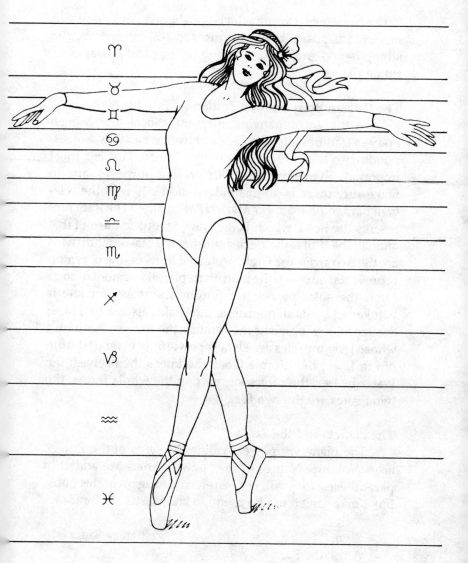

to the planetary powers which are aligned with them. For magical purposes, however, the zodiacal current can be strengthened and "toned" at any time by the power of its ruling planet.

The Human Body and the Zodiac

As the accompanying diagram shows, the human body is traditionally divided into twelve sections, corresponding to the twelve signs of the Zodiac. This is a most important chart relating to our present purposes, and to make sure there is no misunderstanding here is the relevant paragraph from *The Magical Philosophy*: "The Ram represents the head, which is the conspicuous feature of that animal; the Bull is the neck, for the same reason; the Twins are the two arms; the Crab, protected by its casing of armor, represents the chest; the Lion, that splendid symbol of solar force, the solar plexus; the Virgin, the waist, for she is betokened by its slenderness; the Scales are the two hips; the Scorpion represents the genitals; the Archer, the thighs, whose long muscles are always powerfully extended from hip to knee; the nimble Goat, the knees themselves; the Water-bearer, the calves supporting the whole frame; the two Fishes are the two feet."*

The Planets and the Zodiac

The planetary powers ruling the signs of the Zodiac are as follows. Names of the "new" planets are added in parentheses: they will not be referred to again in this book, but it may sometimes be useful to know their attributions:

Sign	Planetary Ruler(s)
Aries, the Ram	Mars
Taurus, the Bull	Venus
Gemini, the Twins	Mercury

*The Apparel of High Magick (Book II of *The Magical Philosophy*) Chapter 1.

Sign	Planetary Ruler(s)
Cancer, the Crab	Moon
Leo, the Lion	Sun
Virgo, the Virgin	Mercury
Libra, the Scales	Venus
Scorpio, the Scorpion	Mars (Pluto)
Sagittarius, the Archer	Jupiter
Capricorn, the Goat	Saturn
Aquarius, the Water-bearer	Saturn (Uranus)
Pisces, the Fishes	Jupiter (Neptune)

The Light Within

It is within ourselves, however, that the magical work has to begin. The forces of the universe surrounding us, no matter how mighty they may be, can only help us to magical power in the measure that we use them as keys to awaken the corresponding force in our inner universe. Then we can use that to act upon the outer world again.

Light, since it is a manifestation of radiant energy, does not only exist in the material world. It is the phenomenon most frequently mentioned by people with inner experience, all the way up through the non-material levels of being: the Astral Light, the Light of the Mind, the Divine Light. You, too, will find and will experience the light of your inner being, both as a lasting joy and source of replenishment, and also as a power you can project outwards for special purposes.

In this present chapter we have gathered the material to form the background for a traditional and potent magical technique which can be of great help to you in the magick of fitness. The method for this follows directly.

Chapter Three

BRING ME MY BOW

Bring me my Bow of burning gold,
Bring me my Arrows of desire!
Bring me my Spear! O clouds, unfold —
Bring me my Chariot of fire!

William Blake, "Jerusalem"

We are stardust
We are golden
And we've got to get ourselves
Back to the garden

Joni Mitchell, "Woodstock"

Each of us needs to be aware of our luminous inner being, and of our Higher Self in particular, for there we have an incomparable source of peace of mind, of confidence, courage and power.

This inner domain is accessible to all, and awareness of it only needs practice and fidelity. You may not find it needs very much practice, for this awareness is a faculty we should have from childhood and keep throughout life, but mostly we have to re-educate ourselves to find it. Fidelity, however, is very desirable. When you once discover the

31

good that this awareness can bring into your life you certainly will not want to give it up, but you may at first need some resolution until a habit is formed, to make sure it doesn't get crowded out of your schedule. Only a few minutes in the course of a busy day are needed to maintain contact.

Contemplation and Action

When you are ready, you can develop your relationship with your inner radiance in many ways, but all these can be classified into two groups.

You can benefit inwardly from your experience of it: being strengthened and refreshed by it, being released from stress and anxiety by the contemplation of it, reexamining problems in that light, being renewed in life and in love. Besides this — and it is "besides", not "either/or" — there are techniques by which you can bring through that light, that radiant energy, to help you in specific ways in the outer world.

Our relationship with outward circumstances is not always happy. Difficulties may be due to things you "can't change" — apparently. They may be due to things you should tackle, but which take energy, resolution and courage; or you may be feeling angry about something, or frustrated or somewhat scared or just plain depressed, and know you are not responding to situations as you otherwise would.

All these things are interrelated with your psychic fitness. "If you want to change the world, start with yourself" — you must have heard or read those words! There's much truth in them. Only (a) the way you need to change yourself is to be more true to yourself, and (b) people who give this advice don't usually offer practical explicit suggestions how to make that start.

Here's one practical and explicit way. You can irradiate

yourself with golden light — golden energy — and with it you can "charge" material substances and things to make them help you be your truer, fitter, more dynamic and effective self.

First Part: the "Inner Work"

1. Stand up. Even if you intend to perform only the "inner work" — as you will while you are learning, and as you may afterwards sometimes for practice, for refreshment or to energize yourself when there is no opportunity for the full procedure — still, unlike some other techniques for bringing through the light of the Higher Self, this one should always be performed standing. However, when you have mastered the visualizations, you will find they are of a type easily accomplished with the eyes *open*: and this can have its own great advantages.

   Drop your shoulders back. Let your arms hang naturally at your sides, then forget them. Your feet should be slightly apart, and parallel. Your posture should be upright, balanced, but relaxed; if you inhale one deep breath and slowly exhale, that should take care of any minor adjustments of alignment.

2. Make sure you are breathing steadily, evenly and fairly deeply. If you are already so accustomed to a form of Rhythmic Breathing that you can do without keeping your attention fixed on it, take up that rhythm now. If you can't do that, this is not the time to begin; simply breathe as if you were in a deep, peaceful sleep. Establish that rhythm, then let it maintain itself while you attend to other matters.

3. Imagine, directly above your head, a sphere of intensely white light, about the size of a tennis ball but very radiant. The exact distance above your

head of this ball of white light does not matter, but, if you have doubts about it, make it about six inches or fifteen centimeters. Visualize it, not as if you were seeing it with your eyes, but as if you were seeing it or sensing its presence and its brilliance with the top of your head. Feel, and realize, this intensely white light, vital and spiritual, pouring down upon you, for it represents the light of your Higher Self.

We work a great deal with visualization but, the way we use it, it is not "make-believe". The light of your Higher Self is really there; your practice of visualization progressively builds a bridge (so to put it) between that spiritual reality and your conscious will. Another analogy: if you have an arm or leg "go to sleep", so as to become altogether without sensation, you exercise it. You move that limb around until its communications are restored and its power of sensation comes back. With it you can now feel the table, the floor or whatever. *But the table and the floor were there all the time.* So likewise the Worlds of non-material reality are there all the time, but exercise may be needed to restore your perception of them. And visualization is an important part of that exercise.

So, before passing on to the next point, linger for a moment with that white brilliance, accepting it, appreciating it.

4. Without disturbing the rhythm of your breathing, on an indrawn breath visualize a shaft of light descending vertically from the sphere of white brilliance to a point in the region of your heart. The shaft is brilliant white, but at the level of your heart the light expands into a sphere of golden yellow light; bright, but not so effulgent at the first.

This is another instance of visualizing something which is profoundly true already, whether you know and think about it or not, and again the purpose of the visualization is so that you can put your imagination and your will into what is happening, thus intensifying its effect in your life.

Your Higher Self is the cosmic "nucleus" of your individual life, of your very existence. The reason why you are directed to visualize the sphere of light which represents it as some distance above your head, not touching you directly, is to emphasize that it is not a part of your "personality". In fact it is divine, and no matter what — absolutely no matter what — might happen in your personal life, your Higher Self could not in any way be injured, diminished or sullied. (That is why, even in extreme trouble, people who are able to raise their consciousness if only for a moment to their Higher Self have always been able to find peace.)

But this cosmic "nucleus" of your being is also the source and origin of your personal life. Hence the direct line of brilliance to your heart — or, rather, to your Heart Center or Heart Chakra — which, itself, glows with a golden fire like sunlight. You are drawing on your inexhaustible cosmic source for strength, love, power and illumination in your personal life.

5. When you are actually performing these actions you should not linger on them, but, as you exhale the same breath which was indrawn in step 4 above, visualize the vertical shaft of white brilliance continuing swiftly down to your feet. You have important Centers in the insteps there (as you have also in the palms of your hands): here you can conveniently visualize the Feet Center as one center of shining,

but not brilliant, white light.

6. On the next in-breath, in visualization draw up from the Feet Center a shaft of fiery bright light, rose-golden in color, to your Heart Center.

7. As you breathe out, be aware of the light remaining in your Heart Center, intensifying the golden light which is already manifested there.

8. Repeat sections 4 through 7, five or six times. Here is a summary of those sections:

   4. Breathing in. Shaft of brilliant white light from sphere above head to Heart Center.

   5. Breathing out. Shaft of brilliant white light from Heart Center to feet.

   6. Breathing in. Shaft of rose-golden light from feet to Heart Center.

   7. Breathing out. Light remains, and becomes intensified, at Heart Center.

After the five or six repetitions of this series, you should be aware of an intense glowing golden radiance at the Heart Center. *If you are doing only the "inner work"*, remain with that awareness for a little while, picturing that radiance, as you breathe, circulating through your entire system — just as you were asked to do with the sunlight in Chapter 2. Be refreshed, restored in courage, made whole in spirit: you are in contact with boundless spiritual goodness and truth, power and beauty, love and peace. Let that contact fill your needs, then let the light of the entire formulation fade from your awareness. Let the Light at the feet disappear first, then the shaft arising from that, and so upwards so that the sphere of white brilliance above the head vanishes last of all.

Second Part: the "Charging Technique"

If you are proceeding with this, perform the "inner work" as above until, after the five or six repetitions of sections 4 through 7, you are aware of an intense glowing golden radiance at your Heart Center. Keep the rhythm of your breathing and, without pausing, continue as follows:

9. Retaining awareness of the three Centers (Crown, Heart and Feet), face — if you are not already doing so — the object you desire to charge with the power you have gathered within you. Focus your gaze upon that object.

10. Raise your arms towards that object until they are extended straight before you, approximately horizontal, then smoothly, in the same sweep of movement, letting the upper arms remain horizontal, flex the elbows and wrists so that the forearms and hands rise higher. In practicing this gesture, the forearm should make an angle of about 135 degrees with the horizontal upper arm: hands are almost vertical, fingers slightly flexed and palms facing front. In actual use, the gesture (which we call the *Orante Gesture*) will naturally be varied somewhat according to the height and size of the object to be focused upon, but the arms should always be approximately parallel to each other, and the four fingers of each hand should be kept touching each other.

    This is a very *natural* gesture of power, and should give you an immediate sense of what you are about to do.

11. Having perfected your focus, maintaining always the same steady rhythm of your breathing, on an out-breath visualize and "feel" the potent golden

radiance from your Heart Center being impelled along through your arms, out through the centers of your palms, and converging upon the object to be charged.

12. Standing again as in section 1, let the light of the entire formulation slowly fade from your awareness, as described at the end of section 8: beginning from your feet, and losing awareness of the sphere of white brilliance above your head the last of all.

Your Sunshine Messenger

One thing needs to be emphasized about this technique. No matter what it is you want to charge, or for what purpose, you always irradiate it with that same wonderful golden light from your Heart Center.

There are ways in which you can very distinctly, and very powerfully, identify and activate the purpose of the charging. These are good, and can give extra force as well as precision to what you do. You will be introduced to some of these methods in Chapter 4, in connection with some specific and valuable chargings you can do for yourself as soon as you have mastered the technique, but in every case you fill your Heart Center with the same radiant golden light, and send that same light forth, no matter in what other ways you "condition" your charging.

Drawing Down Power

Another matter you should specially notice in this technique is the way you build up your available power by repeatedly bringing down the white brilliance from your overhead Crown Center. True, the power you send forth has to be sent from your "personal" levels of being and directed by your conscious will, else you could not "condition" it to your conscious purposes. In this, as in all else, your action should be the balanced and focused act of your whole being, but you should not deplete yourself thereby.

That is a very important general principle. The sending forth of light — energy — from the Heart Center through the palms of the hands is used in the context of many different techniques, most of which have far more elaborate methods than the Charging Technique just given: procedures for healing, for solemnly consecrating a talisman, to give a person or a thing a special dedication, and so on. But always this same central principle holds good: you don't, except in dire emergency, use just your personal energy. It is less powerful, and it leaves you depleted. If there is just a moment to spare, utilize it in bringing down a shaft of light from your Higher Self.

Of course, the more practice you have, the more swiftly and effectively you can do this.

Also you should realize this: supposing, after performing a charging by the method given in this chapter, you find that you do feel a little tired afterwards? You possibly may, if you haven't yet perfected the "inner work" or you are not doing a sufficient number of repetitions of sections 4 through 7. You can attend to those matters at your next performance or practice. Meanwhile, the problem can most likely be easily dealt with by repeating the "inner work" a few times *after* you've performed the charging. If you feel you need to look further for the answer, Chapter 5 should give you the necessary pointers.

The high probability is, however, that no such thing will ever happen to you, and you'll feel that as well as having charged the object you intended, you are also still fully charged, invigorated and in great spirits yourself. That's the way it should be, and most usually is.

Your Homework

Chapter 4 will give you some further techniques and procedures which can be used in connection with the Charging Technique given above. By all means go ahead and read Chapter 4 to see some of the good things there are in store for you, but don't begin the practical work therein until you can fairly competently practice the simple Charging Technique as you have it, without looking at the book.

You do sometimes see people working with power with a "book full of markers". And it can be effective. But, be assured, people with that kind of ability could do real wonders if they'd free themselves from the flipping back and forth and really get into the spirit of the action!

Chapter Four

AY, AY, O AY, . . . A STAR
WITHIN THE MERE . . .

Ay, ay, O ay, the wind that bends the briar—
A star on high, a star within the mere:
Ay, ay, O ay, a star was my desire
And one was far above, and one was near.

Ay, ay, O ay, the wind that bends the grass—
One star of water was, and one was fire
And one for ever shines and one will pass—
Ay, ay, O ay, the wind that moves the mere!

Tennyson, Song from "Idylls of the King"

Part One: Water as We Know It

Water is wonderful stuff: wonderful for its strength, for its receptivity, and for some very curious qualities besides. Also you can, and should, drink it.

From water we draw life, health and fitness. With water we can magically and psychically enhance those benefits. One of the most curious things about water, however, is a plain scientific fact which merits some reflection.

The Strange Case of the Floating Ice

If you heat water towards its boiling point, like any

41

other substance similarly treated its density decreases, it expands; and if you cool it down towards its freezing point, its solidifying point, it shrinks and becomes denser. All that is perfectly normal. But then if you go on lowering the temperature and freeze the water to ice, as it solidifies it suddenly expands again, loses density.

That loss of density on becoming solid is almost unique. Think of the casting of metals, the molding of wax candles; almost any cooling substance goes on becoming steadily denser into the solid state. The only other substance to have come to notice which *sometimes* behaves as water does, is a kind of volcanic glass. When that natural glass expands on solidification, the end product is called pumice; when it solidifies under conditions of pressure which prevent it from expanding, it is called obsidian.

Because water behaves as it does, if people don't take care in cold winter weather they get burst water pipes. But also because water behaves as it does, we still have liquid water on this planet. If water became denser on solidifying, ice would sink as it formed. Since water is a poor conductor of heat, the submerged ice would for the most part never melt. As this effect would be cumulative, we can only conclude that in those circumstances this planet's whole water supply would, many ages back, have become irrevocably frozen up in the two polar ice caps and their extensions. This planet would have been unable, therefore, to support any life "as we know it", as the more cautious scientists say.

Since we *are* here, however, let us take a brief look at some of water's intrinsic properties, and uses for fitness, before considering how you can add further to its powers for yourself.

Formula versus Reality

Early on, we are taught that water is represented by the

formula H$_2$O. Later, however, we realize that water as it comes is inadequately represented by that formula. In daily life water, like truth, is "hardly ever pure, and rarely simple": but luckily our bodies did not evolve in pure H$_2$O, and don't need it now.

Your drinking supply may have additions of fluorine and/or chlorine. The chlorine is only added as a disinfectant, and if it hasn't done its job by the time you come to use the water, then it never will. Consequently there is no reason why you should not get rid of the chlorine at that stage if it bothers you. Boiling will drive off a lot of it, or you can buy the materials to filter it out.

The evidence is that fluorine when imbibed in drinking water really does help cut down on dental decay as it is meant to, although of course it cannot do the work of important nutritional factors. Should you however suspect that the fluorine may be irritating your skin, then either (if just the very sensitive skin of your face is affected) you might simply avoid using the fluoridated water on that area, or else seek medical help.

Apart from those additives, the water supply normally has mineral or organic factors which make it either hard or soft, and either acid or alkaline. It is worthwhile to know what you have in your area. Hard and soft water have different advantages which you can make use of, and you can compensate for their disadvantages in various ways. Broadly speaking, hard water with its high mineral content tends to be proportionately alkaline, good for the teeth and bones, while soft water tends to be acid due to organic influences, is excellent for washing — being kind to the skin and requiring usually a lesser use of soap and detergents — but is lacking in minerals.

All the same, even if you need to soften your local water for washing or to supplement its mineral content in your diet, water is one of your great allies.

Water for Drinking

You probably don't drink enough water, and you probably know that you don't. Naturally, the amount you drink must be governed by your physical capacity, by the nature of the rest of your diet, by the nature of your work and exercise, and by the temperature and humidity of the air. Admitting all these variables, four pints of water a day is a good quantity to aim for. Six is recommended for weight loss programs and by beauty culturists, but, if you want to go for the six, don't worry about it until you are happy with the four. If you want radiant fitness, however, be adamant for the four!

Break the amounts up. If you aim (you may not at first manage it) to drink a pint of water on getting up in the morning, the second pint divided into several small amounts around mid morning, the third pint divided into several small amounts around mid afternoon, and the fourth pint late evening, that will be a very good pattern to establish. You should not, you observe, drink with meals. General custom notwithstanding, if you disrupt the efficient action of your gastric juices by drinking water with meals, you are doing no good thing for your figure, your skin, your digestion or your nerves. (If you feel you must drink something at a meal, drink milk. In fact, that is an excellent time to get this very good food into your schedule, and it can then be digested along with the rest. More on the subject of drinks, foods and stimulants in Chapter 8.)

One of the problems people have with drinking water is that they don't find it "interesting": no matter how good they know it is for them, it still lacks motivation and attractiveness. You can to a great extent take care of this by varying the way you take it. A clear glass of cold water can be very attractive on a hot summer day, and you certainly would not be "cheating" if you were to add a dash — *a dash* — of lemon or lime juice. But you don't have to drink your quota of water all cold and clinical out of a glass all the time. If you feel happier drinking it hot, out of a mug, that's just as good for you and in some ways better. As a matter of fact a lot of wise people these days are quietly drinking a mug of hot water while their friends drink coffee, and there have been instances where half the company is drinking hot water before they realize they all share the same healthful "secret".

Indigestion?

Incidentally, many people find that for an occasional attack of indigestion, a cup of hot water — as hot as they'd drink coffee — is an effective way to quick and lasting relief. The popular "antacids" with which some folk dose themselves *ad lib.* have a real disadvantage: the amount of antacid taken may counteract more than enough of the stomach's natural acid, the stomach then produces more than enough acid to counteract the antacid, and the unhappy owner of the stomach has all the pain and misery to deal with over again. The usual reaction is to take an even bigger dose of antacid . . . etc.

The cup of hot water, which simply dilutes acid instead of attacking it chemically, is for a lot of people the common-sense old "home remedy", even when they know they've well and truly earned their indigestion. Kinds of indigestion which fail to respond to hot water may well be looked at medically, not the least advantage of which is that the sufferer gets a regulated dosage of whatever is prescribed.

As for interest and motivation for drinking water, the latter part of the present chapter should provide you with a good supply of incentives for now and the future!

Water for Swimming

One of the best ways you can apply water to yourself externally is to swim in it. After all, there are not many sports which give you the chance to exercise actively, and to be passively massaged all over, at the same time, but in swimming you can do just that. You can exercise your muscles against the pressure of the water, but at the same time the water is lifting a lot of your body weight so the exercise is less fatiguing; while that same gentle but insistent pressure and movement of the water with its cool tireless fingers is continually massaging, soothing, toning and streamlining your skin and muscle structure.

Because of this double action the benefits recorded from "swimming pool exercise" are astonishing, even in the case of non-swimmers, and even in the case of people who wanted to get back into shape after years of sedentary life.* That is taking into account the physical level alone; when the psychic level of being is considered, there is the beneficial effect of the smooth, repeated rhythms of swimming, the mental relaxation induced by the even support of the water, and the deep instinctual awareness, more profound than any conscious emotion, or return to our primal element. These things are true also of non-swimming water exercise to some extent, for the density of water imposes its own steady unhurried rhythms of movement and gives its own special sense of support and protection.

For the swimmer, however, there is likewise the "encapsuling" nature of the activity itself. The concerns and anxieties of one's land life are for the time being irrelevant. In the world of water another function of the psyche, the Deep Mind, is able to come to the fore: one is wide awake, yet the state of consciousness tends to become altered to something one is otherwise usually able to enjoy only in the sleeping state.

Water for Showering

Showering is a marvelously refreshing and invigorating "toner". As with swimming, there is again a massaging

---

*"Tone up the Swimming-Pool Way" by Curtis Mitchell, in *How to Keep Fit for Life* (The Reader's Digest Association, Inc.)

action; this time, the brisk wake-up tapping on your skin of all those forceful little water drops. Nor is that all: as a less obvious but very real "bonus", the water which is forcefully sent forth in the shower is *negatively ionized* just as is the air you get from an ionizer.

That word "negatively" does not imply anything adverse. It is used strictly in its electrical sense, and negative ionization — whether of air or of water — is a real energizer. Putting it briefly, the atomic and molecular structures of these very fluid substances, such as air and water, are not too closely knit, and numbers of their electrons — tiny charges of "negative" energy — tend in conditions of stress to become detached from their place in the atomic patterns. When the air or water is sent out forcefully in streams from an ionizer or a shower, the molecules thus sprayed forth form themselves into short chains, little "darts" of air or water. Each of these "darts" becomes magnetized, and draws to itself some of the free electrons, which stay with it just for the duration of the "ride". The whole little "dart" thus carries an extra electrical charge, and if you breathe the air or shower with the water you get the benefit.

The Japanese have another angle on showering, and make their characteristically logical recommendation. If you wish to take a cleansing bath, they say — to wash off perspiration, road dust and so on — this should always be done by means of a shower. Send all the impurities down the drain as quickly as possible. The tub should be kept for soaking clean bodies in clean and perhaps herbalized water, for certainly what the body is immersed in will to some extent be drawn into the system.

For Nimble Legs
   The number of beneficial uses for water is almost endless. There is, for instance, the use of alternate hot and cold water to give relief in a variety of conditions, including,

traditionally, sprained ankles and, currently, various minor forms of headache. But one more use of water must be detailed: a favorite with nurses, air hostesses and other busy people who rely very much on their legs. For tired, aching, "heavy" legs, they recommend standing in cool water and splashing the legs with cold. A shampoo spray might be used for the "splashing", or a small mop with a handle, of the kind sometimes used for washing dishes. The essence of it is to refresh the legs with a series of small superficial cold shocks, concentrating on the fronts of the shins, the backs of the knees or wherever else relief might be needed, and to do this daily.

Part Two: Water as Instrument of Power

Enough has been said to show how, even at the directly physical level, water can be used to give immense help in fitness to the entire body, inside and out, head to foot. But in all these uses of water, and in many more, we can step up the power for fitness of even the simplest practices to an immeasurable extent, by —

(a) engaging the action of the Deep Mind, and
(b) invoking effectively the related cosmic energies.

Two Tremendous Power Sources

Make no mistake in your estimate of the two power sources here accessible to you. They are dynamic and immeasurable.

In the major countries of the world, important and extensive researches are going forward into the hidden faculties of the human psyche. These researches are being sponsored not only by universities but also by governments; not for the purpose of finding out whether those hidden faculties exist but, acknowledging their existence, for the purpose of exploring their potential and their mode of operation: telepathy, healing, prediction, psychokinesis and the rest. So far, only the surface has been scratched, but as the work goes ahead and the perspectives become clearer, the sheer power of the Deep Mind (that unconscious part of the emotional-instinctual level of the psyche, from which these hidden faculties come into manifestation) and its ability to control and direct matter, far from being explained away by the investigations, stands out in more wonderful certainty.

Meanwhile, the physicists have met the psychic researchers more than half way. While the direct action of the psyche upon matter by means of directed energy has been demonstrated in many ways, it has also been shown that what is manifest to us as "matter" is entirely built up of negative, positive and neutral charges of *energy*. There is no problem of "bridging the gap" between the psychic and the material levels of being; the phenomenon of energy bridges that gap already.

Your Deep Mind, then, possesses abundantly the power to influence your physical body for radiant and lasting fitness. The remaining question before us is to find means to motivate and direct it to do so.

In emergency conditions your Deep Mind, if you haven't discouraged it too thoroughly, is likely to take action without waiting for your rational consciousness to direct it. We often need help from our Deep mind, however, in circumstances where we have consciously decided what is required, but no profound emotional-instinctual sense of emergency is present.

Mind Over Matter

A few examples will help make clearer what is meant. To begin with, there are the "emergency" type happenings which make news now and then. One time, it was a woman who lifted a car clear of her baby. Another time it was a man who lifted a car and saved a child's life; that feat, also, was plainly beyond the rescuer's muscular strength. Another time a quarryman lifted a huge boulder which had fallen and trapped a companion; one false move, and the trapped man would have been crushed. In such cases, the rescuer when questioned can only say something like "I saw what I had to do, and did it" or, "I only knew I had to act at once". The Deep Mind took charge, and the person's whole psychic and bodily being acted as one unity. It may well be in such cases that the body just goes through the motions spontaneously, while the real action is performed by a kind of *psychokinesis*.

We can compare this with an equally extreme, but planned, exercises of psychic power. Many could be chosen, including firewalking, instant healing, the power to deflect bullets. Fairly recently, a TV feature showed a Yogi who lay down in front of the cameras and supported with his body a wooden runway, over which a twenty-ton truck than passed. The fact that his body did really take the weight of the vehicle was unmistakeably authentic, and he stood up evidently none the worse afterwards.

That Yogi impressed at once by his obvious inner unity of being: psychic power and superb physical fitness were manifest in a harmony which only comes, one knows, when the Higher Self holds the balance.

Your Need of the Cosmic Powers

The example of the Yogi is simply cited as an example of what can be achieved. You, in pursuit of radiant fitness, do not need and presumably do not desire to emulate such a feat. None the less, to produce the results you desire lastingly at phsyical level — for them to be more than a fleeting impression — you do need likewise to engage all the levels of your psyche.

That is where the cosmic powers can help you, and specifically, those great forces which we call the Planetary

Powers. You will have found reference to them in Chapter 2. Primarily these Powers represent divine attributes, divine modes of expression or of being: Justice, Mercy, Beauty, Love and the rest. In polytheistic systems, these attributes are represented by separate deities, whether using the Roman names which we have for the heavenly bodies themselves (such as Jupiter, Sol, Venus) or the Greek (Zeus, Helios or Apollo, Aphrodite) or Babylonian (Marduk, Shemesh, Ishtar) or others. In monotheistic terms, they are all attributes of the One God. It was the Babylonians, however, who first linked the God-forces with the planets, seeing a correspondence between each quality induced by the heavenly bodies, and one or other recognized attribute of divinity.

That correspondence is not surprising. We could hardly recognize, or name, attributes in the Divine Nature which were entirely lacking in human nature:* and in fact each of the planetary powers, reflected in the human psyche, has its own archetypal counterpart in the profound depths thereof. The presence of those deep archetypes corresponding to the planetary powers has been recognized by the most penetrating thinkers through the centuries; in earlier times in Alexandria and the Arab world, later by Marsilio Ficino (one of the principal makers of the Florentine Renaissance and thus the inspirer of much subsequent European thinking), and in the present century by Carl G. Jung (again, one of the makers of the way of thinking of our age.)

In fact, the qualities of the planetary archetypes within the psyche and working through its different levels, make up the main framework of human personality.

Powers Above Us, Powers Within Us

By invocation of any one of the planetary powers,

---

*Except when we conceive of a human quality, and then either magnify or negate it: as omni-potence, im-mutability.

therefore, we invoke in the first place some particular aspect of the Divine Mind; and thus, since like responds to like, we affirm, and awaken our realization of, the presence of our Higher Self which belongs essentially to the World of the Divine. At the same time by making that same invocation, we also stir the archetypal counterpart of that Power in the depths of our psyche, and thus engage our Deep Mind to give power to the work we intend.

There are many ways of invoking and of stirring the planetary powers, and there is much to be gained by studying them; but here they represent only a part of our concern. When we think of the psychic aspects of fitness, we must think of the great influence which the astral world has upon the physical body, and of the strong influence of the Zodiac in the Astral Light. If the planetary powers are mighty in the psyche, it is the zodiacal signs which most greatly influence the body; and as we wish to govern the body through the psyche, we must avail ourselves of the rulership of those signs by the planets.

The Charging Technique Applied

The Charging Technique given in Chapter 3 is basic. In it you have a procedure which need not, and should not, be altered, no matter what you want to charge or how you want to condition the force. It does, however, require additions of one kind and another according to the purpose for which you want it. That is why you should understand and learn the basic technique before adding to it.

Soon you will see how to charge a substance with zodiacal and planetary forces. In this instance the substance charged will be water; for one reason, because water is by nature so great an ally to our life and to our life processes, and for another reason, because water easily transmits any power given to it, just as it easily transmits electricity. (If we wanted to make a permanent talisman, for instance, we would use a more suitable substance and would add more procedures to the charging than we shall add here, which would partly be for the purpose of *locking* the invoked power into the substance.)

What Power-charged Water Can Do

You can thus charge water to the benefit of any part of the body, or, indeed, any function of the psyche. It is not, of course, medicinal, but it can be of very great help in bringing through and augmenting the powers of your Deep Mind to enhance your fitness.

Even where deception has been practiced, and even where it has been a question of real sickness, the instances have been unnumerable through history and into current times, where sufferers have really recovered or improved markedly in condition as soon as their negative mood is cleared away by some action being taken, some attention being bestowed, so their Deep Mind with its immense powers can come through and help them. In contrast, in what you will be doing here there will be no deception, and you will be charging the water yourself with the appropriate powers, by time-honored traditional means. By doing this you will be activating both your Higher Self and your Deep Mind to help you, and at the same time pinpointing just the kind of help you want and expect.

Putting the Power You Want Where You Want It

Most physical culturists know, these days, the value of "focus" where enhancement is desired. It is generally realized now that if you want, for instance, to strengthen or firm the muscles of your arms, you will in any case get results by using suitable exercises, but you will get better results faster if, while doing the exercises, *you focus your attention, with as much positive feeling as you can muster, on the exact muscles you want each exercise to improve.* That method, in fact, is practically essential for some muscles such as Triceps, which, if not "watched", will certainly try to evade their responsibilities.

All that is fine. But, you can very usefully keep the attention of a part of your Deep Mind focused upon your arms even while you are not exercising. (Unlike your conscious mind, your Deep Mind can attend to a number of matters simultaneously and — generally — quite separately from one another.) You need to put through an effective message that this is what you want, and you can do this by charging water for Mercury-Gemini, the details of which you will find further on in this chapter. Then bathe your arms with the water. It's a good idea to have the water rather colder than you would ordinarily wash in, to bring your nervous system into the awareness that something special is happening; and you might use this procedure on alternate days, during the time you are specially exercising your arms.

Supposing a man is aiming to have a taurine neck, or a woman aspires to the kind of firm and queenly column which is ascribed to the "ox-eyed Hera", the same method, of suitable exercise plus bathing, is used with invocation of Venus-Taurus. Both neck and arms afford examples, too, of something else you can do if you wish: the fluid which is charged doesn't have to be water, and you might prefer to charge pure olive oil, for instance, and use it to massage the bodily parts in question.

In many of the good uses of water which have been mentioned in this chapter, whether for internal or external use, you can dynamically enhance its value to yourself by charging it appropriately as a preliminary.

Some Special Cases

The Swimming Pool suggests a few interesting questions: "Hey, I can't charge a whole swimming pool of water.

And what power do I charge it with to benefit my whole body?"

You might be able to charge a large volume of water, though in ordinary circumstances this would mean doing without such accessories as lamps and colored covers (see below). As an alternative, you could charge a small bottleful of water at home with the "full rites", and sprinkle it in the pool. However if observed, this might cause you to be suspected of some unidentifiable kind of antisocial action. The best plan is probably to sprinkle your charged water in the tub at home and take a bath in it, preparatory to swimming.

As to what power to use for charging, Jupiter is the most suitable, bearing in mind that Neptune, deity of the whole waterworld, is really Jupiter's "other self". Don't use Jupiter-Pisces as you would for a footbath, best just use the planetary power of Jupiter and let it permeate the whole of your body from your psyche.

Also, don't be tempted to invoke the planetary power of Neptune for this purpose. Planet Neptune is, as they say, a "higher octave" of Jupiter, and does not relate to the body, but to the world of dreams and visions. If you should be practicing, for instance, to "dream true", that would be the right kind of circumstance for you to charge some water for yourself with the planetary power of Neptune, and drink it. In such a case the God name, lights, and color to use would be the same as are given below for Jupiter, but the Sign visualized would be that of Neptune. (See the list of planetary uses which concludes this chapter.)

"Toners" for the Psyche

If you want to charge water to enhance some faculty of your psyche, then charge it for the appropriate planetary power only, and drink it. If you want to charge water for a bodily benefit, but not to limit its power to any part of your body, use the planetary power alone; in such a case you have the choice whether to drink the water or to bathe with it. The power of Venus for beauty, for example, or of Mars for strength, if implanted in the psyche will certainly take effect in the body.

"If my doctor prescribes a bottle of physic for me, may I step up its psychic helpfulness to me by charging it with the power of Mercury?" — Yes, but the doctor-patient relationship should not always be a one-way thing. If you do what you suggest, it may be helpful to you, but have mercy on your doctor's blood pressure and say nothing about your action!

Now to the details of how the tables below should be used.

Preparing to Do the Charging

You need to know that you are not dependent on the accessories. To learn to judge between essentials and inessentials, and in various emergencies to be willing to "improvise or do without" not only makes you a more effective and helpful person in life generally, it also advances your spiritual evolution. You learn, in fact, to appreciate and to use whatever resources are available, without tying them around your neck.

At the same time, the Deep Mind undeniably likes accessories. Machiavelli, that hyper-shrewd analyst of human behavior and motivation, was in his working life a pen-pusher in a minor post which did nothing for his self-image. He tells of his great delight, after a day at the office, to return home, take a bath, change into a magnificent robe and sit down for a quiet evening with the classics. He pursued his studies not as a clerk but as a scholar, and his genius flourished accordingly.

As any week-end painter discovers, too, the attic or garden-shed studio has to be kept ready for *the artist* to walk into. Once the equipment with its rich clutter of colors and smells is stashed away in a closet, the thread of imagination and inspiration gets broken and is difficult to re-join.

The best attitude to adopt, then, in matters relating to psychic fitness, just as with other activities which involve the Deep Mind, is that of *the serious player.* While one corner of your awareness knows your Deep Mind certainly has the power to keep you radiantly fit by itself, you are also conscious that by doing everything as properly as you can, you will be signaling unmistakeably to your Deep Mind that you mean seriously what you are doing. The preparations will thus also involve every level of your being directly with the action. All this is important.

Your Working Area, and Yourself
You will need to use a small table, or part of a large one; the small table is preferable. You will also need enough space so you can stand back from it. If in the early stages you want to have this book near you, or a paper with your own notes for the exact charging you intend, keep them right away from your working table. For one thing, this is physically more orderly. For another thing, if you do have to consult the papers at any point, you don't want any doubtful or hesitant vibes of "What do I do next?" getting projected into your good work. Keep the papers right back where you will be standing: have a reading stand, or a music stand, or a chair for the purpose, or, if you are using a single sheet of paper with your own notes, stick it on the wall with a bit of tape.

Don't hang it on a cord around your neck or wrist. Certainly you see people equipped in that way at the kind of ceremony where everyone makes speeches and nothing much is done, except maybe the sun rising which happens of itself. What you are about to do is essentially *practical.* When you do the actual charging, if anything is dangling from neck or wrist it is liable to dip in the water or to topple something over, or else so much of your attention may be taken up by ensuring this doesn't happen that the charging itself is done less than singlemindedly.

The same sort of care should be taken with what you wear. If you have a special "meditation robe" or something similar which is neutral in color — white, black, gray or "natural" — you may wish to wear that when you perform a charging. That is good, and is one of the things which can help give that important signal to your Deep Mind to come in on the proceedings. But if your robe happens to have long, wide sleeves, don't just be optimistic but pin them right up to almost as high as your elbows. One large safety pin per sleeve will do it.

If you don't have a special garment, then wear whatever is clean, comfortable and neutral in color. If you can be barefoot, do, otherwise an easy-fitting but secure pair of sandals, slippers or sneakers will serve.

You yourself should be bathed and tidy, and it's good if everything you wear can be freshly laundered. Your working area should be free from irrelevant objects of any kind (but no need to move heavy furniture, pot plants or aquaria) and freshly dusted and polished. Clear your mind from clutter too; take a few minutes to relax physically and mentally and to detach yourself from whatever you have just been doing. *Even stop thinking, for this time, about the reason why you want to charge this material.* You simply intend to charge it.

Charging with a Zodiacal Influence and its Ruling Planetary Power

(1) The Zodiacal Influence

The zodiacal influence is represented by the zodiacal sign and also by a "color charge". A very good mode of introducing the zodiacal color is as a piece of fabric (such as felt) or paper on which the material to be charged can stand. Rectangular pieces of felt or paper in many of the colors listed below can often be obtained at stores which sell supplies for school projects, and you can build up a collection over a period of time.

If the color charge is employed in that way, the zodiacal sign should be drawn in black on a white card. If the above method of employing the zodiacal color is not practicable, the zodiacal sign may be painted in its zodiacal color on either black or white card, whichever will show it to best advantage. In that case, the material to be charged should be placed upon either black or white, at choice.

In all cases, liquid (such as water) to be charged should be contained in colorless transparent glass. The card, on which the zodiacal sign should be drawn about 3 inches or 8 centimeters high, should be securely set up (as on a bookrest or in a photo frame) a little distance behind the material to be charged.

In the list below, the colors shown in capitals are to be exact spectrum colors (again, educational supplies should have no difficulty with these). The other colors are relative to these, and any color which answers the description may be used. "Yellow green" for example might be "spring green", "linden green", "mistletoe green" etc: "green blue" might be "teal" or "prussian blue", etc. Always to be avoided in this work are heavy, confused shades such as loden green, plum purple or yellow ocher.

In a very real sense, this is an *alchemical* work: the colors, signs and materials you use at the physical level form as it were the meeting place where your will can encounter, and can direct, the spiritual forces. You can make this encounter all the stronger and more intimate as you select, handle, work upon, and employ your own mental powers in relation to the physical materials.

Zodiacal Table

Name of Zodiacal Sign	Zodiacal Sign	Zodiacal Color
Aries	♈	RED
Taurus	♉	Red orange
Gemini	♊	ORANGE
Cancer	♋	Orange yellow
Leo	♌	YELLOW
Virgo	♍	Yellow green
Libra	♎	GREEN
Scorpio	♏	Green blue
Sagittarius	♐	BLUE
Capricorn	♑	INDIGO
Aquarius	♒	VIOLET
Pisces	♓	Magenta

(2) The Planetary Power

The planetary power is much more strongly represented than the zodiacal influence. Not only is the planetary power the ruling and directing force, it has also to call forth, and to carry, the response of your psyche: of your whole psyche, spiritual heights to unconscious deeps.

The planetary power is represented in this charging by:

> *The Lights.* It is necessary that these should be of the correct planetary *number*, as shown in the table below. Votive lights in transparent containers are preferred, but candles may be used. They should be placed on the table behind and around the material to be charged, but not where they will be in the way

of the charging. Or they may be placed around the area of working, none of them then being on the table. They are to be lit prior to the charging.

The *color* of the lights — that is, of the outward transparency through which they will shine — should be of the correct planetary color as shown in the table below: that is, as nearly as possible to the true spectrum color.* If however you cannot obtain a sufficient number of the correct color, you must use the right number of colorless transparent ones. The entire planetary number must be uniform. The same rules apply to candles, although those of course only give white light in any case.

The God-name. This is to be uttered aloud at the first moment of sending the power through your hands in the charging.

While it must be said that the use of a God-name is optional, it is very desirable, so that the power invoked may engage all levels both cosmically and in your psyche. The Hebrew God-names which correspond to the planetary powers are given here as being very potent, ancient, and acceptable to most Western people. If you know and prefer to use other divine names, and if you are certain of their correct correspondence to the heavenly bodies, then certainly you can substitute them.†

---

*Votive light holders in red, green, blue and yellow can often be had, and violet may be found in appropriate stores at the approach of the Advent and Lenten seasons, but amber may have to stand in for orange, and smoke grey for indigo (which should, rightly, be a deep blue that inclines neither to violet nor to green). Or you may get lucky and locate a do-it-yourself kit for dipping electric bulbs for Christmas or carnival, in which case you'll obtain colorless transparent votive-light holders and dip them every color you want.

†In Western usage, the Roman names of the deities have for centuries been too closely identified with the planets themselves to have much force for many people: you are not advised to use them as deity names, therefore, unless the Roman deities really mean something vital to you personally. For many people the Hebrew names have a greater sense of "specialness" and so a greater power. If, however, you would prefer instead of the Hebrew names to invoke the names of the Roman, Etruscan, Greek or Babylonian deities associated with the planets, these, with notes on their nature, attributes, and special functions and concerns, will be found in "Planetary Magick" by Denning and Phillips. (Forthcoming from Llewellyn).

The Planetary Signs. These also are given in the following table, but they are not for material representation in your area of working. If, however, you wish to draw them large for the sake of impressing them clearly on your memory, that is an excellent idea. As you prepare to do the charging, you are to visualize the planetary sign, to identify the controlling planetary power of the charging, at the mental and astral levels of being. (The God-name you will utter identifies the power at the divine level, the lamps identify it at the material level.)

Planetary Table

Name of Luminary	Planetary Sign	Number of Lights	Color of Lights	Divine Name for Invocation
Saturn, Uranus	♄, ♅	3	Indigo	Yah-veh El-o-him
Jupiter, Neptune	♃, ♆	4	Blue	El
Mars, Pluto	♂, ♇	5	Red	El-o-him Gi-bor
Sun	☉	6	Yellow	El-o-ha Va Da-ath
Venus	♀	7	Green	Yah-veh Tza-ba-oth
Mercury	☿	8	Orange	El-o-him Tza-ba-oth
Moon	☽	9	Violet	Shad-dai El Cha-i

The divine names in this list are divided so as to help you give each syllable its full value, not stressing one part of the name at the expense of another. To try to represent these ancient names with pedantic accuracy would be out of place in context of a language with such variable and complex vowel sounds as English. If you can speak Spanish or any other continental European language, it will help you a lot here. Otherwise, just pronounce the names as they look, but *generously.*

In the Sun name, keep the two syllables of Da-ath separate. Properly, you should if you can close your throat for an instant between the a's: this is known technically as a "glottal stop". In the Moon name, the Ch is a guttural — between "k" and "h".

If, when performing any charging, you can pronounce the appropriate divine name in a chanting or singing voice, that's glorious; but if not, just say it loud and clear.

How it all works out

At this stage the whole procedure may look complicated, but in reality it isn't; particularly if you have already mastered the basic charging technique in Chapter 3. After all, on any given occasion you'll only be using those zodiacal and planetary correspondences which relate to the specific charging you then intend to do. That is why it is a good idea, when planning a charging, to copy out the details you need on a separate sheet of paper. Let's take an example.

Breasts Like the Full Moon

The women of the island of Bali have, as their traditional costume, a kind of sarong which leaves the breasts bare: and they have always been noted for their beautifully shaped, firm, high breasts, whether in early girlhood or mature matronhood. Also as a matter of long tradition, they have attributed this lovely distinction to their custom, from childhood onwards, of splashing their breasts daily with cold water.

Now, supposing a woman of standard Western upbringing resolves to improve her figure in the manner, and by the method, of the Balinese tradition.

To offset the relatively late start and to enhance the value of the water-splashing, to maintain her interest in it and to gain the help of the dynamic powers of her psyche and of the cosmos, she decides to use charged water for the purpose.

(She doesn't need to charge a bowl of cold water every morning. She can charge a bottleful, and add a dash of it to each day's splash-bath.)

The appropriate charging (see Chapter 2) is *the Sign of Cancer ruled by the Moon.*

Assembling the Materials

(See, first, the Zodiacal Table in this present chapter.) Maybe she doesn't find any orange-yellow paper of fabric, so she mixes together some orange and yellow paints, such as poster colors, and paints the Sign of Cancer on a stiff piece of black paper because that will show the color well. She puts the water she means to charge in a clear glass bottle on, maybe, a white cloth on a small table, and sets up the card behind it. That takes care of the zodiacal part of the preparation.

Now for the planetary part. (Look at the Planetary Table.) Let's say she has taken an opportunity to provide herself with nine violet "Advent lamps". (They'll be good for many more chargings than this. This chapter concludes with a list of uses for different planetary chargings.) There may not be room on the small table, so she places them on chests, window ledges, etc., around her "working area". Now, having lit the lamps, she is ready to begin.

The Lunar Charging

She proceeds with the Charging Technique exactly as in Chapter 3, up to the point where she has just raised her hands in the Orante gesture. There she pauses for a moment and, not losing awareness of the golden light at her heart center, she visualizes, calls to mind as clearly as she can, the crescent Sign of the Moon. The color is not important, she can visualize it in black and white. Then, keeping if possible awareness of that sign (but in any case she has now *put it there*, astrally) she projects from the palms of her hands the light from her heart center into the bottle of water, pronouncing as she does so the divine name "Shaddai El Chai".

She will remain thus for a moment to realize and affirm

what she has done, but the charging is now complete.

Using a Planetary Power Alone

The only reason why this needs to be described is to reassure you that it really is as simple as it looks. Supposing someone wants, for example, to reinforce their courage; either as an ongoing program, or for a special occasion. Unless they really are getting "butterflies" badly in the solar plexus, there is no need to bring in the physical level with the zodiacal sign of Leo. Simply refer to the Planetary Table.

Our friend places a transparent colorless glass of water centrally on the table, on a square of black or white fabric or paper. Maybe votive lights were not available, or maybe our friend likes doing psychic work with candles, so six yellow candles are set up around the glass.

The Charging Technique proceeds exactly as in Chapter 3, until, while the hands are lifted in the Orante gesture, the Sign of the Sun is visualized. Then, with the projection of the light from the heart center, comes the utterance of the divine name "Eloha Va Daath".

The charging is complete.

The Force Is With You!

No exhaustive list could ever be given, either of uses of water charged with both zodiacal and planetary powers, or for those charged with the planetary powers alone. What is sure, however, is that the entire technique and use of psychically charged water is available for each person to use and apply, according to his or her own will and inclination.

To conclude the subject, here is a list of suggested uses to which you could put water charged with a planetary power alone. Since no specific part of the body is involved, these would be simply for charging and drinking. *To your psychic health and fitness!*

The Planetary Powers

Saturn (ruler of Capricorn)—For patience, perseverance; for the help of the Deep Mind in projecting a more mature or dignified self-image; for use when working to improve memory, concentration, attention to detail; for inner self-control, sense of economy. To open the door to awareness of one's Higher Self.

Uranus (ruler of Aquarius)—To enhance one's sense of adventure, for the help of the Deep Mind in detaching oneself from unwanted emotions, breaking the grip of the past; to discover new perspectives, and to be aware of flashes of creative or inventive insight.

Jupiter (ruler of Sagittarius)—For optimism, enthusiasm, generosity. For use when cultivating one's consciousness of life's abundance, as when preparing for Creative Visualization. To gain the help of the Deep Mind in projecting a more genial self-image, especially where one is in a position of authority or seniority.

Neptune (ruler of Pisces)—For use when seeking development of psychic faculties, particularly those which relate to dreams, visions. For heightened appreciation of music, painting, poetry; for development of talents relating to the media.

Mars (ruler of Aries)—For alertness, enterprise, energy. To gain the help of the Deep Mind in developing a more positive and assertive attitude, especially when one has been conditioned or habituated to self-effacement. For use while acquiring skill in handling tools, instruments, weapons of any kind. To gain the help of the Deep Mind in running, wrestling, boxing, winter sports or any ball game; also for energetic forms of dancing such as many ethnic dances.

Pluto (ruler of Scorpio)—For help in all solitary, private or secret projects where the aid of other people cannot readily be sought; also in meditation. To enlist the power of the Deep Mind for psychic recuperation, whether after sickness, financial loss or any bad news. For use also when employing one's personal magnetism in a public situation.

Sun (ruler of Leo)—To enhance one's psychic energies in general; to gain clarity of purpose and inner equilibrium; to gain the help of the Deep Mind and the Higher Self in acting in a more enlightened way, and thereby to project a nobler self-image, inspire loyalty in others, attract friendship. Also for spiritual and psychic protection.

Venus (ruler of Taurus and Libra)—To enhance one's esthetic sense in general, to gain the help of the Deep Mind in projecting a more sensitive and romantic self-image; for the positive attitude which attracts luck, rewards; for help in developing the decorative arts, in entertaining, and in the more graceful and feminine modes of dancing. To enhance one's attractiveness. For harmony and beauty.

Mercury (ruler of Gemini and Virgo)—To gain psychic power for improving one's faculties of communication, whether in conversation generally, especially in all-over "aliveness", vibrant intercommunication between body and psyche.

Moon (ruler of Cancer)—To gain the help of the Deep Mind in increasing one's appreciation of, and capacity for, sexual love at both the emotional and physical levels. To enhance one's sense of humor and power of fantasy. To overcome a tendency to laziness or procrastination. For help to develop one's ability to understand, educate, or take care of children. To strengthen relationship with one's own Deep Mind, as when preparing for Astral Projection. To enhance psychic powers for psychometry, dowsing etc.

Finally: Don't think of these chargings as something for use only in emergencies. Charge water often, often drink, or bathe with, psychically charged water. Besides the inner strength, help and protection you gain as a result, it is good for you often to perform the chargings themselves, often to fill yourself with the light of your Higher Self. And, the more you do this, the greater light and power you will be able to draw down.

Chapter Five

COME WITH BOWS BENT

Come with bows bent and with emptying of quivers,
  Maiden most perfect, lady of light,
With a noise of winds and many rivers,
  With a clamor of waters, and with might:
Bind on thy sandals, O thou most fleet,
Over the splendor and speed of thy feet
For the faint east quickens, the wan west shivers
  Round the feet of the day and the feet of the night.
  A.C. Swinburne, Chorus from "Atalanta in Calydon".

Of the things most essential and most supportive to
our life, we have considered somewhat of Light and Water.
Next we may well consider Air — "Wild air, world-mother-
ing air," as is necessary to our life, more air to our good
health, and more air still is every way desirable for our
abundant and radiant fitness. "Like a breath of fresh air" —
"A healthy outdoor complexion" — nobody ever needs to
explain these phrases: they represent something we all understand, an acknowledgment we all make.

The canoe, kayak, raft or yacht enthusiast, the backpack-
er, trekker, rock climber and camper in their season, are
doing much for their fitness in face of a way of life which

69

otherwise, for many people, threatens to become as shut-in as the age of the four-poster bed. But not everyone has the opportunities they would desire, and, in any case, although vacations and weekends can help you through the year very beneficially, there may still be ways in which (a) more air can be brought into your daily living, and (b) your psyche can be involved to enhance the worth and power of your physical activities in this regard.

Your Breathing is Not Done For You!

Someone might say, "Why do we humans have to bother about our breathing? — why can't we just do it spontaneously as the animals do?"

The answer is, *Not all the animals breathe quite spontaneously, and we happen to be related to some that don't.*

It is fairly common knowledge these days that we are to some degree related to those wonderful creatures, the dolphins. We, and they, can trust to the autonomic (not governed by the conscious will) nerves to maintain breathing even when we are paying no attention to it, once the breathing habit is established; but baby humans quite often, and baby dolphins always, have to be forcibly started to acquire that habit. Baby humans are customarily put on the right track by means of a slap on the buttocks; baby dolphins, by being held right up out of the water by their mother and her companions. It is the adult dolphins, not the infants, who instinctively cope with the situation. (That, incidentally, is why dolphins will support above water any creature they find helplessly floundering therein. Some "authorities" have stated that the stories of dolphins saving swimmers in distress were only legend or fable — presumably because they themselves never saw it happen — but it truly does happen, and here you have the reason why the dolphins do this. The helpless creature appeals to their instincts as being a newborn of some kind.)

From the beginning of life, therefore, breathing is not entirely spontaneous, and we have plenty of evidence in human experience that, despite habit, breathing remains as it were uneasily poised between the spontaneous and the deliberate, between the domain of the autonomic nerves and that of the cerebro-spinal (conscious thought) system.

Did you ever have the rather unpleasant experience, when you got thoroughly engrossed in something, of unexpectedly giving a sort of choking hiccup? — because, without noticing it, you had stopped breathing until your air-starved lungs prompted you to start up again? It not uncommonly happens to people. It is one of the reasons why the Yogis train their pupils in good habits of regular breathing, so that their deep meditations may not be interrupted by any such disconcerting accidents.

However, even at that we are better off than the whales, who have to breathe quite deliberately, and would stop completely if they ever lapsed into sleep for more than a few seconds at a time. The whales show every sign of a rich joy in living in the world of sensation, but if our breathing were as theirs, surely we should lack the sublime realms of thought and, probably, also of dream?

Helping the Way you Breathe

The fact that this essential life process, breathing, has both unconscious and conscious controls is of great value to us in improving the quality of your breathing. You can consciously exercise yourself in good methods and patterns of breathing, and although you cannot dictate to your unconscious mind — your Deep Mind — that it shall adopt the same methods and patterns when it is in charge of your breathing, you will find it very easy, with a bit of perseverence, to make these good ways attractive to your Deep Mind and to habituate it to them.

Overcoming the Negatives

There are four main reasons why people breathe inadequately: bad posture, bad programming, stress, and laziness. (Here must also be mentioned another reason, not a "main" one but one which unfortunately affects quite a lot of people: trying to avoid a continual bad smell. This might be of industrial origin in your workplace, or it might be from the cigarettes of people around you in an office, for instance. In such cases you probably have a legitimate cause of complaint, but unless or until you can get the situation put right, you have the choice either of removing yourself from it, or of ensuring that out of working hours you get as much good air into your system as possible.)

The four main reasons all have to be dealt with by means of one area of your body: your diaphragm.

Your Chest is an Accordion

Air does not go into, or leave, an accordion because the middle portion of the instrument actively draws it in or blows it out. The drawing and blowing effect is present, but only because the instrument is extended or compressed from the ends. Imagine holding an accordion vertically, with the upper hand stationary and the lower hand doing all the work, and you have a fair model of the way your lungs are operated, or the way they ought to be operated. If for any reason your diaphragm is not taking care of the action properly, you are not breathing adequately. (Your diaphragm is a more-or-less horizontal sheet of muscle, at the level of the base of the breastbone, forming a "floor" to the chest and a "roof" to the abdominal cavity.)

Faulty posture is one cause of the trouble: sitting your knees too high or your shoulders crouched forward, so that your middle is cramped in, or even with your body habitually twisted around from the waist to manipulate some piece of equipment. Only you can know whether you need different seating arrangements (a cushion on the chair may be all that's needed) or better lighting, or maybe your eyesight needs some help. Another problem occasionally met with is that a person feels self-conscious about adopting good posture. Fortunately that attitude is getting much scarcer since more robust types are finding favor in fiction once more. That's an example of "programming".

On the subject of programming, a little needs to be said about a particular example. It isn't many years back that once, when I was talking about the function of the diaphragm in breathing, somebody said to me, "But you're only talking for the men. Women don't breathe that way!"

A Harmful Myth

It may be that some women still breathe without very much movement of the diaphragm. This is a breathing defect known as "high chest breathing". It not only deprives the body of its proper quota of air but it is also bad for the lungs themselves, parts of which may never get properly expanded and exercised. This defect can beset not only women, but also young men if they have been studiously inclined or for any reason sedentary from boyhood. The reason for the "selectiveness" of this faulty way of breathing is simply that it *can* only affect people who have slender, flexible ribs.

No matter how flexible your ribs may be, however, you can and should train yourself to breathe from the diaphragm. Of course, numbers of women these days do so quite naturally. High chest breathing may have its uses at some stages of pregnancy, but if so, when it is necessary it will develop naturally. All the more reason why a woman should give herself the benefit of healthy breathing (which means also healthy blood) during all the rest of her life.

The notion that women do, or should, breathe in a basically different manner from men is usually attributed, and probably rightlly, to the tight-lacing tradition. It may be a number of generations since any woman in a given family went in for tight-lacing, but still, in many families, generation after generation of daughters have been programmed to the effect that in breathing, as in many other things, Mother must be their model. Remember, this kind of "family programming" is at the emotional-instinctual level, and therefore largely unconscious unless and until you dig for it, and Mother is often the model and ideal for the daughters, not only because they love and admire her, but also because she presumably represents Father's ideal too. On those terms, a piece of bad programming, such as that of high chest breathing, can not only survive through a number of generations, but can sometimes be the subject of unthinking emotional defence.

If your ribs are flexible, of course they will lift to some extent when you inhale; so they should, but the main movement should be in the diaphragm. If you happen to be a habitual "high chest breather", a good plan is to place the palm of one hand across your upper chest, and the palm of the other hand across the space where your lower ribs part company just below the breastbone: and then breathe in slowly and deeply, keeping the higher hand as still as possible (this is just an exercise) but making sure to push the lower hand out with the muscles of your upper abdomen. Then, as you exhale, relax and let both hands resume their original positions. After some practice with this, you'll get the feel and the habit of diaphragm breathing, and can stop this exaggerated practice.

In case the men who keep their ribs completely rigid think they are 100% right, let them be assured they too may be able to improve their breathing; but before going on to that, let us finish dealing with the cramped diaphragm. The next two causes of trouble affect men and women alike.

Tension: Your Diaphragm is a Muscle

Stress, tension; everyone has experienced it at some time or other. You might be lying in bed, going over some problem in your mind and wondering why you don't go to sleep and forget it until morning, when you realize maybe that instead of resting, every muscle in your body is tense. Or you may be watching an exciting movie, and suddenly realize you are no longer sitting in the relaxed, easy posture you had at first, but that all your muscles have tensed up as you follow the action.

Tension is usually the result of a situation, real or imaginary, which seems to call for action, but in which, for whatever reason, you are powerless to act. Therefore, before you resolutely relax your muscles, it's a good thing to give them something to do. Either you can progressively flex as tightly as possible, then relax, every set of muscles in your body in turn, or a tussle with a favorite piece of exercise equipment, or some exercise without equipment, is also to be recommended. After this exercise, of course relax progressively and as completely as possible.

In such practices, it is important not to neglect the diaphragm. Not only is the diaphragm a muscle, but, perhaps because of its proximity to the solar plexus, it is particularly liable to be affected by nervous stress. For that reason, in moments of acute emotional pressure, people often instinctively defend themselves by standing or sitting upright, quietly, and for a minute or so taking no notice of what may be going on around them while they take a succession of perhaps three long, slow, deep breaths, in and out. This is usually very effective in restoring inner calm and allowing a fresh view of the situation.

It is better still, if that cramping-up of the diaphragm can be avoided by its habitual exercise in the practice of steady, deep, rhythmic breathing, such as will be given in this chapter. These exercises are not only physically good, they help prevent tension also by psychic means: building inner strength, confidence and stability.

Laziness and Procrastination

Little needs saying about laziness. Lazy people usually know they are lazy, and they generally stay that way until something changes them. Well, now this book has come along and it should give everyone some good motives for action.

An insidious form of laziness, however, which frequently keeps people from realizing how lazy they are, is *procrastination:* the talent for never doing today what can be put off to tomorrow. What is deferred to tomorrow, no matter how favorably it is regarded, often doesn't get done at all.

The mail order advertisers know this, of course, which is why they always urge, *Rush your order off to us today!* In such cases you will often do well, on the contrary, to think the matter over for a day or so. But in the present instance, where nobody stands to gain or lose but you, don't make hollow promises to yourself. Having read this book through once, go through it again, decide upon the practices you immediately need *and start in without further delay.*

Unless you already have an established breathing exercise (and even if you have, for an additional method can be useful) you should include at least one from this chapter.

"Stone Walls Do Not A Prison Make"

—but cast-iron ribs can. They can make you feel depressed, frustrated, misunderstood. They can deplete your physical vitality and your self-assurance. They can lessen other people's image of you, and consequently their opinion of you.

Which is meant here is the opposite breathing defect

from the "high chest breathing" which was mentioned as being mostly a problem for women. This might well be called "No chest breathing", and is mostly a problem for men.

Just occasionally a woman has something like this problem; usually someone fairly young, who has a well-developed bust and is shy about it. Now, a good bust is nothing on earth for a woman to be shy about, but the thing to do, if she feels like that, is to get a "minimizer" bra. Then she can stop hazarding her health and well-being by trying to maintain a collapsed-looking chest, and can re-learn good breathing habits.

For men, learning or re-learning good breathing habits takes more effort because of those less flexible ribs. What is needed is to habituate your ribs to lifting so as to give space for you to inhale more air, and to re-train and tone your diaphragm into doing its rightful work.

The diaphragm, already described as being more or less horizontal in the body, is normally domed upwards somewhat into the chest. If it loses its "tone", it can sag downwards into the abdominal cavity, thus causing the bulge in that area which is associated with a flat chest.* But remember — the diaphragm is a muscle. You can re-train it, just as the biceps or any other muscle can be re-trained after neglect.

For a Better shaped Chest with More Air Capacity

For most practices — including breathing practices — which can be performed while seated, we recommend a straight-backed chair on which you can sit with spine vertical, thighs horizontal, the legs from the knees down vertical, and the feet parallel with both heel and toe resting on

---

*An abdominal bulge can be due to various causes, and more than one cause can be present: a sagging diaphragm, simple external fat, displaced or ailing internal organs, spinal weakness. If in doubt, or if pain or tenderness occurs, medical advice should be sought.

the floor. This is the "Egyptian Posture". (If you don't find a chair which is just right for you, you can of course make adjustments with cushions, footrests etc.)

For this particular practice, however, you need a slightly different arrangement. You can use just the same chair, but in this case place in front of it a footstool, box or so forth about eight or nine inches high, on which you can place your feet securely. Torso and lower legs alike will still be vertical, but now your thighs will not be horizontal, they will slope up from your body to your knees. This brings your abdominal muscles into more effective play.

This is one of those exercises in which you need to follow in imagination what is happening inside you to be able to direct it properly. (That, in fact, is good advice for any exercise.)

1. Being seated as described above, begin to inhale as slowly as you comfortably can. You should be able to feel the air filling the lower part of your lungs, pressing against your lower ribs.

2. Still inhaling, by your imagination and your will "direct" the air higher up, first to the back and then to the front of your lungs.

3. Complete your inhalation, in the same way "directing" the air to fill the top region of your chest cavity. Then, while holding your breath, proceed *at once* to the next section (prolonged holding of the breath without monitoring is undesirable).

4. As strongly as you can, contract your abdominal muscles. Make an effort to pull in the diaphragm area too. This will have the effect of pressing the inhaled air upwards, compelling your upper ribs into action, and at the same time giving your diaphragm some beneficial activity.

5. After three heartbeats, exhale.

After one or two natural breaths, repeat the procedure.

Don't overdo this exercise at first, but practice it twice a day, aiming to work up to 25 repetitions at each session. As with every physical exercise which is worth doing at all, the virtue lies in the quality of each repetition rather than in sheer number of repetitions.

Bear in mind, moreover, that this is only an exercise. You are not trying to re-train yourself to contract your abdominal muscles every time you inhale; that is only an "emergency measure" to get some lift and expansion into your upper ribs and some "tone" into your diaphragm. Other times, breathe naturally — *but make use of your increased breath capacity.*

For Everyone: Benefit to Psyche as well as Body

Now that everyone — hopefully — has the knack of breathing with the diaphragm and making use of their real lung capacity, the next step will be to try some different forms of Rhythmic Breathing.

Since our breathing is a special and practically unique kind of activity in the functioning of the body, in which, as we have seen, both the conscious mind and the unconscious — the Deep Mind — plays its part, *the act of breathing provides us with a special and valuable "common ground" which our conscious mind can use to communicate with the unconscious areas of our psyche.*

This fact is recognized in both Eastern and Western teaching. In the terse and austere language of the *Hatha Yoga Pradipika,* which is meant to be meditated upon rather than to be completely comprehended instantly, it is said, "When the breath stirs, the mind stirs also." Nor is Yoga the only system in which it is recognized that by means of the breathing, powerful suggestions can be passed to the psyche. There are examples in the Far Eastern discipline of Tao, and in the Western world — particularly in the Byzantine and allied traditions — examples both historical and modern can be found of controlled breathing used as a potent vehicle for mystical prayer.

As you will be shown, you can use rhythmic breathing to assist your progress in many ways, both physically and in your psyche.

Two Types of Rhythmic Breathing

Although just two types of rhythmic breathing are given in this section, in each one there is considerable flexibility as to the actual timing to be employed. The object is for you to find the exact one which is, for you, the most congenial, and then to practice it until it becomes second nature.

When you have chosen a *type* of breathing for practice, you are likely to find after some time that the *timing* you initially chose is no longer right for you. That is to be expected, and you may find there are several such changes, progressively, until with the established habit of better breathing you find your true norm. If after trying one type you come to the conclusion that you chose the wrong one, then by all means change. Both types are good, and traditional. But do settle to one or the other as soon as you can.

When you can practice your chosen type and timing of breathing for a considerable period deliberately, give yourself this test. Start off your rhythmic breathing, then immerse yourself in some absorbing activity. Forget about your breathing for, say, half an hour, then check to see if you are continuing in the established rhythm. Then test yourself with an hour. You should reach the stage, in time, when you can lie down to sleep at night, establish your rhythmic breathing with a resolve to continue it, and awake to find you are in fact still breathing in the same rhythm. That takes time and patience, but it is a good objective.

The "Healing Breath"

The first of these two types of breathing is known to a good many people as the "Healing Breath". It is called that because its habitual use generates a great deal of free-flowing energy, which is one of the chief things a healer needs to be able to give, but we generally recommend it to anyone who wants to prepare for any type of psychic activity. The pattern of this rhythm is 2-1-2-1: that is, breathe in for a certain number of heartbeats,* hold the breath *In* for half that number, breathe out for the same number as for breathing in, and hold the breath *out* for the half number.

The effect is rather like the rhythm of breathing which establishes itself naturally during peaceful sleep, when the whole system is steadily replenishing its energies. You might breathe in during six heartbeats, hold the breath for three, breathe out during six and hold the breath out for three. Or you might make it eight, four, eight, four. Or perhaps four, two, four, two, just at first.

In any case, notice that this is to be an easy form of breathing, without any straining. You are not meant either to overfill your lungs, or to empty them completely.

The "Pranayama Breath"

As its name implies, this is a traditional Yogic method of drawing *prana* — life force — from the atmosphere, so it too is suited for fitness. This method has no pronounced pause between the out-breath and the next in-breath, so there are only three groups of heartbeats to count. For beginners, the pattern is 1-2-2; that is, if you breathe in dur-

---

*Some authorities recommend counting by seconds. We see no reason for setting up such a deliberate conflict with one's natural rhythm.

ing two heartbeats, you are to hold your breath for four heartbeats, then to breathe out during four heartbeats, breathing in again during the next two heartbeats. When proficiency in this is acquired, the pattern should be changed to 1-4-2; that is to say, if two heartbeats are taken for breathing in, the breath is then to be held for eight heartbeats and exhaled during four. This is strongly in contrast to the method of the Healing Breath, where the pattern never changes although the number of heartbeats used will change with practice.

In fact, the "Healing Breath" and the "Pranayama Breath", although both are of Oriental origin, are completely in contrast to each other. Each has its natural adherents, and you can discover which you prefer. Many other forms of rhythmic breathing have been devised by teachers both Eastern and Western. Some are meant for use on particular occasions, and of many it can be said that you should only adopt them if you mean to understand, and follow, the particular philosophy with which they are associated. They are too specialized to have place here.

Good Applications for your Rhythmic Breathing

Because all good things are available to us in the astral, mental and spiritual levels of existence — depending upon what kind of good things they are — then it is not fiction, but a good piece of creative affirmation, if we inwardly "see", and draw to ourselves, the benefits we desire with the air we breathe. From quite early in your practice of your Rhythmic Breathing — as soon as you can to any extent leave it to your Deep Mind to maintain it while you give your attention to something else — you can use that Rhythmic Breathing to convey messages to your Deep Mind. These will not be messages in words, which are not the Deep Mind's preferred form of communication, but messages in picture, in emotional tone, in sensation. These messages will be very well received, assimilated, and acted upon.

If you feel you need to surround yourself and fill yourself with a particular color, either to express your inner feelings or to compensate for something lacking, you can do it this way. Sometimes one feels a great "hunger" for a particular color. Establish your Rhythmic Breathing, close your eyes, imagine, feel, know yourself to be surrounded with a brightly luminous astral cloud of that color. At every in-breath, draw it deeply into yourself through your lungs, through your pores.

You can take that a stage further. Whether you have a physical colored light, or have evoked it for yourself astrally, you can affirm, "With this yellow light I draw in clear perception, understanding..." or "With this red (or orange) light I draw in energy, stimulation, strength . . ." or "With this green (or blue) light peace, harmony, inner oneness . . ." and feel the quality pervading you, restoring you. This is really another "charging technique". You can charge yourself with a color for the benefit of others, too. If you want to go further into this, get a book on color and the wonderful things it can do.*

Also, with practice, you can build up something more complex and let your Rhythmic Breathing carry it powerfully into your Deep Mind. You can, with closed eyes, build up around you, really experience, "breathe the air of", any place or time of present or past that appeals to you; with such reality, by this method, that this present time and place can seem almost unreal when you return to it! Or you can build into the future. Do you have some cherished personal wish or daydream? With your Rhythmic Breathing, eyes closed, go forward into the time of its fulfillment. Leave behind all anxieties, all poignant longing concerning it, and relax in the radiant peace of its realization. That way, you'll

---

*Such as *Practical Color Magick* by Raymond Buckland (Llewellyn).

not only have a happy experience here and now, you will be helping strengthen the reality of what you are affirming in the astral world, helping "materialize" it for its future earthly fulfillment.

You may want to go forward into, and so help bring to earth, that future time of which Tennyson wrote a century back,

"When the war-drums sound no longer, when
the banners all are furled,
In the Parliament of Man, the Federation
of the World."

We should have more people dwelling upon (literally dwelling *In*) that, to help outbalance all those others who, from no matter what good motives, are trying to fill people's view of the future with visions of doom and destruction. *That shall not be!*

Or, do you love animals, trees, green growing things, fair rivers? You can — and should — build up a "garden of Eden" in the astral. It will not lack for innocent inhabitants.

With any of these "wish fulfillment" visualizations you build up in this way, it's a very good thing to conclude by visualizing above your head the brilliant white light of your Higher Self, as described in Section 3 of the technique in Chapter 3. Then bring a beam of white light down from it to illuminate the whole astral scene around you. See it getting brighter and brighter, with a wonderful sense of joyousness and peace. At last you can't see the scene for the dazzle of white light, but you know it is all still there, more real than ever. Then, gradually, let the light too fade from your consciousness. You can, of course, continue your Rhythmic Breathing as long as you wish.

Bringing down the light of your Higher Self in that way is really a very powerful way of saying "Amen" or "So may it be".

Breathing With Your Skin

No matter what good pure air you breathe into your lungs, or how much you improve your capacity for doing so, you still need to breathe through your skin.

The manufacturers of clothing for outdoorspeople know this. The more effective garments become in shutting body heat in and adverse weather out, the more thorough the insulation, the more we find them designed with zippered turtlenecks, zip-out sleeves and so on, giving the wearer considerable ventilation at a moment's notice.

You may remember, in Ian Fleming's *Goldfinger*, the episode of the young woman who died because her skin was covered with gold all over. Certainly that was fiction, but other instances have occurred in real life. Probably the first time it was realized — after the event — that the complete coating of the skin was somehow responsible, was at a sumptuous pageant in medieval Italy, when a boy covered with gold to represent Cupid collapsed and died.

This is also one of the main reasons — apart from shock and possible sepsis — why a person with extensive burns is always regarded medically as being in a dangerous condition; the damaged skin has lost its power to breathe.

In terms of your general fitness, all this means that your skin's need to breathe has to be respected. It means such things as "sauna suit" methods of slimming should be very restricted in their use. It means, on the beach, that relaxing in semi shade with a lightly protected skin is of more benefit to you than lying in full sun covered from hairline to toes in heavy goo.

It also means that although swimming and bathing in water is most excellently good for you, it ought not to be the only kind of bath you take.

Bathing in Air

These days, more and more people seem to have less

and less opportunity of taking off their clothes in a natural way in their own homes. But some good opportunities are missed, too, through mistaken interpretation of example.

Perhaps, mornings, you watch on TV teams of young women and men, all in very good shape, bouncing on their toes in front of the cameras as they do aerobic dances or exercises. Maybe you join in with them — a marvelous toner.

Of course the main idea is to increase the amount of air, and thus of oxygen, breathed into the lungs. But, with that type of exercise, you can take the opportunity to aerate your whole body too, breathing in more air through your skin. It all benefits your blood, your heart, your whole system. To take full advantage of this, however; don't be tempted to think that because the people on TV look so good in their complete suits of tights you ought to wear the same. They are on a public show, you aren't. If you want to wear something special, why not a swimsuit?

Other times, such as when you get up in the morning — just after your tub or shower for instance — see if you can let there be a few minutes' interval between taking off your robe and getting into your daywear. Same thing, in reverse, at night. You may at those times be doing nothing but sit or stand, but you'll soon feel your skin appreciating its breath of freedom.

But there are other types of costume which give your skin a wonderful chance to breathe, and in which you can indulge in some very healthful activity besides. Many such styles — gauzy flowing skirts, loose-fitting oriental trousers, bikini-type outfits, fly-away scarves, shawls, brief bolero jackets, take your choice — are traditional to the magnificent, individual-expression art which is generally known as "belly dancing", but which Daniela Gioseffi has in these days well named "Earth Dancing".

Again, the subject is too big to be treated effectively

here:* but to numbers of women, and men too, the acceptance of this joyful, expressive and natural mode of dancing as a part of American life has opened inspiring new vistas of purpose, of artistic creativity and of well-being. Even to those who do not aspire to make "Earth Dancing" a regular hobby, it gives a new impetus and incentive to express themselves spontaneously in dance when they feel like it.

Dancing with the Elements

Dion Fortune, in her book *Psychic Self Defence,* tells of a glorious, wild and completely spontaneous experience into which she and some friends were suddenly caught, one day on a sunlit, windy hilltop. On an impulse, Dion raised her hands in invocation, and at that moment — equally on impulse — another of their friends came rushing up the hill to join them. Suddenly they were all dancing, with no pre-arrangement and no conscious co-ordination at all, but, Dion Fortune tells us, she realized every person was dancing sunwise, turning on their own axis as well as in a general circular movement as a group.

Everyone who gets to know the inner nature, the intimate "feeling" of the elements, agrees that Air is the wild unpredictable one, untameable and sometimes even tricksy, but unequalled for vitality, for the zest and joy of living. Let it into your life, breathe it into your body and into your psyche, and be strong!

Eliminating the Negative

Let's admit it, the circumstances of our lives are not always all sweetness and light, and we ourselves aren't all sweetness and light either. Human beings in general are liable to all kinds of negative feelings, including sheer blazing anger at the negative attitudes of others.

---

*See *Earth Dancing,* by Daniela Gioseffi (Stackpole Books).

What can you do if you find yourself in the grip of some kind of negative emotion? The first thing, certainly, is to see if there is some kind of action you can reasonably take in the matter; whether to find allies in righting an injustice, or to improve your self-image if you have been slighted, or to direct everything to a goal whose importance to you you've just realized, or to seek new interests, or whatever seems to fit the case. If you can take any action at all it is likely to release some of the tension and help you feel better.

But however you cope with the situation, in many cases there is likely to be a residue of bitterness, a "bad taste in the mouth" which just has to be gotten out of your system. And here, if you have acquired the habit of individual dancing, you have a good method ready to hand.

If you can do this outdoors, that is better. If by chance you can use the occasion of a strong breeze, that's better still. But if you have to build up the open country scene and the whirling wind in your imagination as you dance — you can do that!

You may be able to put on some helpful music, such as Grieg's "In the Hall of the Mountain King", or, for a real hurt, Saint-Saens' "La Danse Macabre". The important thing is that you should be able to let yourself go, to give expression to all those negative emotions, to dance them truly out. But — and this is the essential thing — as you give these emotions forth, you must feel the winds taking them; not merely freeing you from them, but scattering them, dispersing them, obliterating them. As you yield them up, they are snatched away and are forever gone. This must be so, whether you are availing yourself of a physical wind or have summoned up an astral one. The dance should leave you clean in a clean world, and ready to take a new grip on life.

And Affirming the Positive

If you take to dance as a form of self-expression — and it's somewhere inside each person — you'll soon realize how much more powerfully you can express your wishes, your hopes, joys and loves in dance. Dance to the rhythm of your Rhythmic Breath, or simply to the beat of your pulse. Dance within the wish-pictures you build up, dance in your Eden or your Utopia. Dance as your breathe in colored light — all the colors of the rainbow together if you so desire — visualize them flashing and swirling around you, as you glide, run, move as you will among them, caressed by them, absorbing them! Of all the earthly elements, Air is the one most like the Astral Light, and it is a means of life. In your own life, realize its potential as fully as you can.

Chapter Six

I AM LOOKING AT TREES

I am looking at trees
 . . .   .
and though I seldom embrace the ones I see
and have never been able to speak with one
I listen to them tenderly . . .

W.S. Merwin, "Trees"

I cannot tell what you say, rosy rocks,
 I cannot tell what you say:
But I know that there is a spirit in you
 And a word in you this day.

Charles Kingsley, "Dartside"

As you become more aware, with practice, of the non-material levels and faculties of your own individuality, so increasingly you will develop the ability to discern and to appreciate some of the life forces, and some of the simple "currents of energy", in the world around you.

This is not so paradoxical as it may seem. Your everyday rational consciousness is in reality the part of your psyche which is "shut up inside" your body with only the five senses as "windows": while, above and below it (figuratively speaking), your Higher Self and your Deep Mind

91

have their own powerful and extensive means of knowledge and of communication. (Only, to be accurate, your
Higher Self doesn't need any "means".) Your rational consciousness is therefore well advised to cultivate close and
friendly relations with these two helpful neighbors.

It has happened several times in history that some
quiet, meditative and seemingly introspective person has
proved to have a more exact idea of what was going on in an
entire country than anyone else, plus a more practical notion as to how the situation should be handled.

"Inner Illumination"

A very good way to encourage and help this development is to establish your Rhythmic Breathing (see Chapter
5), then to bring down the light of your Higher Self, building it up as in Chapter 3, sections 3 through 8; but when you
have brought it to as much intensity as you can in your
Heart Center, then become aware of it irradiating your
whole psychic and physical being.

You only want to "seal", by invocation of this supernal
light *on to it*, the astral image of something you *truly desire*. In
the present instance, your purpose is simply to perceive
what is, so we have this different procedure of bringing
down that light at the beginning of your practice, in order
for you to learn to "see" by it and in it.

(Don't be misled by that word "see". On the one hand,
"seers" frequently not only "see" visions, but "hear" voices
or other sounds, "smell" odors both sweet and repellant,
and "feel" various sensations including changes of temperature. On the other hand, the whole experience can be
very abstract and "mental" and you may receive a vivid
impression of scenes without "seeing" them or of words
without "hearing" them. Those matters are very individual.)

Imagination, the Learning Aid

When you are practicing using these inner faculties, don't be afraid to use your imagination. Quite a lot of people are held back by that fear, and by nothing else; while, in fact, using your imagination gives you excellent opportunities to train your inner faculties.

You can compare this training with the way, for instance, young children are generally taught to use their outer-world faculties and abilities. When a child is learning to count, whether workbooks or instructional toys are used, there is something of a conceptual barrier between those things and the world of everyday life. The toys, like the images in the book, lack a certain quality of "reality" because they exist only to be counted. And, quite often, one sees a child deliberately and triumphantly crossing that barrier, looking up suddenly from the workbook or the learning game, gazing around and saying "There are six chairs in this room!"

Just as important as the comprehension of counting is the realization into which that child has just stepped, that counting is not just for grouping colored beads correctly or seeing how many balloons the artist has drawn. In the same way your inner faculties may very well develop among images created by your imagination. One day they will begin to contemplate the wider non-material worlds, and you will find their true perceptions impinging on your consciousness.

What people mostly fear, of course, is that they may mistake their early "practice" imaginings for reality. Generally they will not, and if occasionally they do so, there is in the vast majority of cases no great harm done. Serious delusions begin at a very different level of the psyche, with some sort of fanaticism, or obsession, which would be sure to cause one kind of trouble or another. The real "danger" with the type of practice we are considering is just the other way around; that you may "see" something real, and think you've imagined it.

Even that is usually of no great consequence, unless you are a writer of fiction. Then there is a degree of possibility that, on account of something you truly think you've created, you may find yourself accused of libel or plagiarism. Or even — as happened to one unfortunate strip cartoonist — of complicity in a modern act of piracy on the high seas!

Don't worry about it. A normal person's imagination does tend to gravitate towards truth, but "seeing in the light of your Higher Self" should give you real help in discerning the difference between what you create and what you recognize as being already "there".

Earth Currents

The world around us is full of tides, currents, energies; influences of every description, including the structures and stresses of the Earth itself.

The causes and effects of some of the great forces operating at physical level are fairly evident, or are becoming progressively recognized as science accepts them and gives names to them. It is often pointed out that giving a name to a force — gravity, electricity — does not explain it. This is true, but a name well given does at least indicate what type of force we are considering, and helps form mental concepts of it which will relate rightly and truly to our mental concepts of other matters. Most creative thinking is done by means of this continual comparing and contrasting of our ideas on different matters, judging how they relate to each other and what that relationship signifies.

Sir Isaac Newton, as everyone knows, pondered the fall of the apple and identified the force of gravity. But, as the great Goethe pointed out, if we inquire how the apple came to be up there above Newton's head in the first place

— the active growing force of the tree from the ground up into the light — we are considering a different kind of force from gravity: a living, perceiving force.

For the moment we are considering the first kind of force. Even these "mechanical" forces, however, can be mysterious enough, and we are surrounded by all kinds of them.

The Big Magnet

Currents of energy which affect everyone to some extent, whether they realize it or not, are those mighty vibrations and rhythms set up by the Earth's double rotation: its rotation around the Sun, and its spin on its own axis.

The axial spin in particular sets up an intense pull to the north, for the north and south "poles" really are the "poles" of the huge magnet which the Earth is by reason of its movement. The north pole not only attracts lodestones and magnetic steel needles: those things are attracted so swiftly and violently that we can see them move and use them for pointers to the north, but the geologists tell us that even the huge land masses which form the continents of this planet are moving northward, slowly but irresistibly; this independently of the widening of the rifts, the sinking of the plains and the other slow changes of which they tell us.

This great and continual north-south tension is part of our lifelong environment, and while — whether sitting or standing — we have our spine vertical, it probably makes little difference to us. When we lie down, however, it can make a considerable difference.

Because of the shape human beings are, you will present less area for the magnetism to act upon if you lie endwise to it instead of across its direction of pull. Also, if anything movable within you (such as your blood) is going to be drawn in one direction, however slightly, it is better attracted towards your head than towards your feet. For these reasons, it looks likely that the old belief is justified, which says that to sleep well you should sleep with your head to the north. Certainly if you sleep less soundly than you should, you would do well to check the position of your bed by the compass and, if you don't already lie with your head to the north, give it a trial.

"Getting from Under"

There is an exception to this head-north rule, and it should be noted here because it shows a little of the complexity of the web of powers around us. Not only are we surrounded by influences from everything around us, but there are some which originate with us also.

Supposing you always sleep with your head to the north, but then a time comes when for some nights, on account of some special anxiety or grief, you find yourself unable to sleep. You seem to have forgotten how to relax, and every time you lie down at night to stare at the ceiling you wonder if you'll ever sleep properly again.

When you feel the time has come to release yourself from whatever the trouble may be, *make up your bed head to foot.* Leave your bed exactly where it is, but put your pillows at the foot end. This is no superstition, no "charm to bring sleep", although it will act like one. If you were clairvoyant, you'd be able to see all the gloomy clouds of negative emotion you have created, literally hanging over the head part of your bed, waiting to descend again on your head, face and solar plexus and to afflict you again when you draw them in.

Sleep the new way round for a couple weeks, more or less, as you feel about it; sleep you will, and the dark clouds will disperse. Then when you are ready, go back to your head-north way of sleeping, all fresh as if from a vacation.

(You can hasten the going of those dark astral clouds.

Charge some water for Sun-Leo and sprinkle just a few drops on your bed from head to foot, every morning just after you get up and every night just before you go to bed, visualizing golden radiance sparkling and streaming from the scattered drops. While you do this, you may like to say such words as:

Sunshine, fill my place of rest:
Night shall bring me slumber blest!

Do this for six days, the solar number in this system. Any of the charged water that's left at the end of this time, drink it last thing at night with a feeling of light and peace irradiating your heart as you do so.)

More Magnets

The Moon is another mighty magnet. It is neither near enough to Earth, nor sufficiently constant in direction, to have any perceptible effect on the land masses, but everyone knows how the more responsive element, water, obeys the pull of the moon in the ebb and flow of the tides. And our bodies are made up about 97% of water. In addition to the power of the Moon's polarized light (see Chapter 2), therefore, we can expect to be to some extent "pulled" by the Moon whenever that luminary is nearest to us, i.e., directly overhead, no matter whether the Moon is visible at night or invisible in the daylight. Are you sensitive to this? Do you sometimes go out of doors at night in response to some unreasoned impulse, and look up to find the Moon is directly overhead? Keeping track of these things is not only fun, an added interest in life, it's also another little piece to add into your increasing picture of self-awareness.

There are other big magnets too, not so large as the Moon, but much nearer. Mountains, and even large buildings, exert quite a measurable degree of magnetism, a "gravitational pull". People who have spend a few years, or more, where there are mountains nearby or on the skyline often feel a curious sense of "something missing" if they go to live at another place, maybe at about the same altitude, but without the presence of mountain peaks or ridges. This need not be simply an emotional lack. As one woman put it, "It's very like the feeling of being without my pack, after a long backpacking vacation: a bodily sense of missing a familiar pressure".

On the other hand, people who are not accustomed to that kind of vertical gravitational pull can find it oppressive, disturbing to the solar plexus, although it may not be strong enough for them to identify the cause of the sensation. This is likely to be a reason why some people feel "threatened" in mountainous (or big-city) environments.

For Psychic Power and Peace

If you have a skyline which is dominated by a mountain or a mountain ridge, or if you have such a scene vividly in your memory or imagination, you can make it the subject of some interesting and valuable experiences in meditation. (Additionally, if you tend to feel oppressed or "over-looked" by mountains, this may prove helpful with regard to that too. If you love mountains, of course, all the better!)

Sit where you can see your mountain straight in front of you, either physically or "in your mind's eye". Ideally, you should sit in the Egyptian Posture and establish your Rhythmic Breathing, as described in Chapter 5, but if these conditions are impossible or inconvenient, then at least you should sit in a balanced, easy but alert posture and breathe in the steady and rather deep manner you would associate with peaceful sleep.

Gaze at the mountain, as you might gaze at a person whose character you wished to study in detail. From its shape, what elements have left their signature there — fire, water, wind? Or, after the water and the fire had done their work, have the slow unmeasurable pressures of Earth conspired, through age after unperceiving age, to thrust this colossal mass up inch by inch towards the skies? However you interpret its history, you can regard with wondering admiration the mighty strength, the endurance and the beauty of the mountain as you perceive it now.

If possible — and even if you are seeing your mountain in memory or in imagination — look at it under several aspects: in the dawn, in the full day, bright sky or storm, by sunset, beneath the moon. Then choose a time, early morning or evening perhaps, when the misty atmosphere has in itself an ethereal, dreamlike quality, for the next stage of your meditation.

Riding the Pull

As you sit breathing rhythmically, looking across at your mountain, image to yourself a fine line which runs from about the middle of the mountain to your solar plexus. This line is taut and there is a slight pull on it, because it represents the magnetic pull which the mass of the mountain exerts upon you; a pull of which you can be aware, but still not too strong for you to be able to choose whether you respond to it or not.

When you are ready, you can imagine yourself beginning to move forward along that line, steadily and by your own volition, towards the mountain. You can appreciate that magnetic attraction for what it is: one among the great but by no means hostile forces of the world, with which you can play if you wish.

So you glide at your own controlled speed towards the mountain. Nearly there, you decide where you will "land". The magnetic line was only a guideline, you don't have to go with it all the way to the central area of the mountain unless you choose. You could equally select any other spot. Let's say you decide on the summit.

Imagine yourself there, gazing across an immense expanse of iridescent sky into the rosy fire of sunrise: a luminous wilderness of colors, which are reflected, fragmented and concentrated changefully in the myriad tiny crystals of the snow about your feet. And the perfection of that snow is not sullied by any footprint of yours. The magnetic pull is not particularly noticeable to you now, since it is a simple gravitational attraction beneath your feet where everyone is accustomed to it. Delight in all the beauty and power of which you partake; inhale it, bathe your inner being in it, make that mighty tranquility a part of you.

(This, incidentally, is a very good preliminary meditation if you are preparing yourself to do true astral projection, training for the out-of-the-body experience. We would not generally advise anyone to make it their first experience of actual projection of consciousness from the body; not that any real harm would be likely to come of it, but just because a sudden quasi-physical realization of the vastness, the height and the solitude could be unnerving until a person has gained some experience of projection. But as an imaginative foretaste of the *feeling* of going forth astrally, it is excellent.)

Another Mountain Experience

For a variation on the above which you may sometimes enjoy as a psychic refresher, let us go back to the point where you are sitting visualizing the magnetic line from the mountain to your solar plexus.

As before, begin, when you choose, to move in imagination along that line, but when you have gone a short distance — again, at your own choice — stop, as if your consciousness were hovering in the air not far removed from your physical body.

Be aware of the magnetic line pulling you, but at the

same time — and, in particular, with every in-breath — imagine that you in turn are drawing from the mountain, along that same line, all the strength and stability, confidence and serenity of the mountain. Fill your psyche with those qualities, to bring them back into your body and into normal awareness.

At the end of either of these meditations, there is no need of any visualization of returning back "along the line". Just let the scene you have built up gradually fade from your consciousness, or, if the earthly mountain is before you, disengage your attention from it. Focus your awareness on your breathing, on the chair where you sit, on the feel of the floor beneath your feet, of your hands resting on your thighs. Continue your rhythmic breathing, at least for a little while as you regain your earthly perspectives.

The Silver Trail

If you are a water person rather than a mountain person — or just for a change, if you are both — you can perform very similar meditations to the two just given, but focusing your attention on that shining track which leads across a calm lake, river or ocean when the Moon shines above. A night of the Full Moon is best for this, but here, too, you can work with the scene itself or with an imagination of it. Likewise, you can go up in imagination to where the pure light reflects so shiningly off the silent Moon craters, or you can go a short way upon the trail and draw into yourself, from the gaze of the Moon, an emotional-instinctual comprehension of the ways of the Astral World, of the mysteries of love, and of the hidden face of nature. As with the mountain meditations, make your return afterwards simply by renewing your awareness of your physical environment.

Your Sensitive Solar Plexus

After reading through the foregoing meditation meth-

ods, you may ask "Why my solar plexus? Surely if a magnetic or gravitational force is acting upon me it must be acting upon the whole of me?"

Certainly that is the case. But the solar plexus, more
than most other regions of the body, is what we call *astro-
sensitive*; that is to say, it responds sensitively to influences
which might otherwise pass unnoticed, whether those influences are physical, emotional-instinctual, or psychic.

Furthermore, it is sensitive in this way in practically all
human beings. There are other astro-sensitive regions —
the back of the neck and shoulders, the soles of the feet for
instance — but they are not effective for everyone, and in
any case they are less conveniently located for most practical purposes.

Naturally, the sensitivity of the solar plexus is shared
by the surrounding bodily organs. Everyone knows what is
meant by a "gut feeling", usually a feeling as to the truth,
genuineness or lastingness of a situation as presented;
while even the most elegant critic is likely to describe his or
her personal response to a painting, a book or a musical
composition as "visceral". If the hands and arms are brought
into the region of the solar plexus, they share in its sensitivity.

You may know of, or have read of, some of the marvelous achievements of *dowsers*, people who can "divine"
the presence of underground water or metals for example,
or can locate lost objects or missing persons. Dowsers, or
diviners, generally use an implement which may be a twig,
a twist of cane or of wire, a pair of metal rods, or a pen-
dulum. Mostly they go over the terrain itself, but some can
obtain remarkable results simply by holding their pen-
dulum over a map.

This matter is dealt with at considerable length in the
Practical Guide to the Development of Psychic Powers, by Denning and Phillips;* on page 180 of that book is a drawing of a

---
*Llewellyn 1981.

young man with a pair of divining rods, and the way he is holding them at the level of his solar plexus is typical of the use of divining instruments generally.

The important thing for you is this: Dowsing implements only *indicate*. The evidence is that they indicate what your solar plexus already "feels", what your Deep Mind already knows, although the feeling and the knowing are at a level which in process of growing up your conscious mind has been trained to ignore. Now — for the sake of your fitness, your health, your nerves, your total radiant aliveness — undo some of that training. Use your solar plexus in meditation, as indicated above. Also "ask" it where you put your keys, spectacles, anything you've mislaid, and give it a chance to pull you in the right direction. Give it time — you probably haven't taken notice of it for years. Pay heed, too, to its voluntary messages — those "gut feelings", "visceral emotions". Let it help you live!

Recharging the Nervous System

Many of us get so little opportunity to revitalize ourselves with anything like a spell of natural life in natural surroundings, that although we may do our utmost with the annual vacation, times spend betweenwhiles in even a small park area can be precious.

Your Rhythmic Breathing is excellent almost anywhere, although you should get right out of the fumes from the highway if you can. To be conscious of inhaling good air purified by the sunshine, or fresh from the hills or from the sea, is a great tonic for the psyche as well as for the body. Fortunately, also, there are two very good methods for recharging, bringing into balance and calming the whole nervous system, and you should be sure to take any opportunities to do one or other.

They can be done magnificently in the open country where you can give ample time and full attention to the practice, alone or with a few like-minded friends; but they will also confer much benefit upon you if performed where time and space are limited, and where maybe children are playing and other people enjoying the fresh air in their own different modes nearby.

For those occasions, it can be added that there is nothing you need feel self-conscious about, or that will particularly attract attention, in these actions. There's nothing strange about a person lying on the ground on a pleasant day, or leaning against a tree. The "secret" is in the special way you set about it.

As the main nerves of your body run off from the spinal cord to branch into all parts of your body, there is all your life a two-way passage of electrical energy along the spine from brain to body, from body to brain. When that energy runs high, you feel "on top of the world" physically and mentally. When that energy runs low, or is impeded — for instance by poor spinal posture — there may not be anything wrong with your *health* exactly, but you'll begin to feel less than 100% good; lacking in brain-body synchronization, lacking in attention, and unaccountably either lethargic or irritable. So here you are going to (a) straighten your spine even more than normal for a short time, and (b) bring in some good electrical energy from an outside source.

Earth Energy

Lie down on your back, your head due North, flat on the grass or the sand, or what have you. If you feel you want a layer of something between the ground and you, that's okay, but try to choose an old-fashioned, "breatheable" blanket and certainly not a "Space Blanket".

Check that you make one straight line from head to heels. Have your heels just about an inch apart. Don't totally relax your feet, keep just enough tension in them to hold the toes parallel. Raise your knees very slightly, to tilt your pelvis slightly up in front and help straighten the mid-region of your back to lie nearer the ground. Tuck your chin in — also slightly — so as to avoid lying uncomfortably on the back of your head.

This is what we call the "Earth Posture". Usually, to complete this posture, the arms should lie straight but relaxed at the sides, the hands with palms naturally inclined somewhat towards the ground but lying limp, partially open with curved fingers. In this case however, there is a variation. The arms lie at the sides, but the elbows are bent just sufficiently to allow the palms to lie flat on the ground, fingers extended and slightly parted so that each finger tip has its Earth contact too. That way, you get considerably more vitalizing Earth contact, also (in case it matters) you look less helpless, less vulnerable than with hands slack.

Lying thus, North to South, establish your Rhythmic Breathing. Use your imagination at first to pick up the great Earth currents flowing through you and pulsing under your hands and your spinal column. Let these currents pervade you, vitalizing and purifying. Picture them continuously flowing up your spine and your arms to your head, then down your two sides and your legs, carrying psychic wastes, negative emotions, away out through your feet.

It is for you to choose how long you will lie thus, but twenty minutes is as much as you should feel you require. With more practice in this type of self-energization, you should be able to gather more power in less time. When you have done, remember to be thankful to our Mother the Earth. She sustains our lives no matter how we act, but in reverent thanks we find a greater harmony with her.

The Strength of the Tree
Just as when taking Earth energy you should be careful to lie head-north, so, before taking tree power, you should be careful in the choice of your tree.

You should seek a large, mature tree which shows no signs of failing strength; but if you cannot find one of that description, then choose a rather younger tree. A mature oak or a redwood is ideal, ash and beech are very good; the maples and sycamores are friendly trees, but do not give forth so much energy, perhaps on account of their high sap content. The elms are, for several reasons, not recommended, and of course you should avoid trees known to be poisonous, such as the horse chestnut. Those with rough or thorny trunks, or the conifers whose branches spring from near the ground, clearly do not wish to receive this kind of attention.

Having found your tree, simply stand with your back to it, straightening your spine against the trunk by slightly bending your knees, as was described for gathering Earth energy. Put both your hands somewhat back from your body, to press your open palms against the trunk at about the level of your hips.

When you are practiced in this you will not need to use your imagination, but at first use it to find the sensation of warm energy almost tingling into the full length of your spine, refreshing and revitalizing you. Remain thus for about twenty minutes, if you so desire.

Before you leave, thank your tree and wish it well. These are not the easiest times for our beautiful gracious friends.

About Talismans and "Luck Pieces"

Many people like to have a "luck piece" or talisman of some sort which goes around with them in pocket or purse, or on a chain or cord at the neck.

There are several different kinds of talisman. There is the kind a person deliberately makes, starting with the right raw materials and building up a type of "psychic magnet" to draw the natural powers and influences for love, prosperity or for some other special benefit. The making of such a talisman is a work in itself, and the subject is too big for this book.

There is the kind of talisman that a person finds, such as a coin — perhaps of no great monetary worth — which by its date, or the time or place where it was found, has a special significance to the finder. He or she doesn't want to part with it, so has a hole drilled in it so as to carry it as a "luck piece".

To the Greeks of old, such a "luck piece" was known as a "Gift of Hermes", a little token of favor from the Messenger of the Gods.

The kind of talisman to be brought to your notice here is rather like that in some ways, but the "feeling" of it, the kind of power it carries, is different, more serious.

The Nature Talisman

As you become more aware, more attuned to the forces and energies surrounding you in the material world, you will be able to "keep an eye open" for your own special Nature Talisman.

The ideas which follow are to a great extent based on Native American custom, but with a recognition of the very similar ideas existing throughout the continent of Africa, and, indeed, wherever people have lived for long ages in conscious contact with the natural forces and have developed their own spontaneous responses to them.

A Nature Talisman is a natural object which in some way attracts your attention, impressing you with the feeling of potent forces being concentrated, or focused, within it. There should also be something about the shape, size, color or the whole "idiom" of its presence, which gives you the feeling that it was waiting there for *you*.

It might be a piece of fossilized wood or even of driftwood, a bit of coral or a seashell, or a fossil of any kind, but perhaps the most likely thing is that it will be simply a rock. If you feel strongly drawn to a rock, but realize it is rather too large to be comfortably carried around, don't be put off. A "pet rock" is a friendly companion, and can be a focal point for good influences, if given a place on your desk or your nightstand. Again, supposing in process of time you acquire several Nature Talismans, any one of which you can wear, but not all? In those circumstances you choose for any given day the one you feel is most suitable. The proper way to keep the ones you are not wearing is in a special bag, pouch or purse, which you should preferably make yourself, but in any case keep strictly for this one purpose. (You can certainly keep in the same bag any other talismans of whatever kind that you have, provided you feel equally positive about each one and have the same sense of personal attachment.)

Besides just waiting for your Nature Talisman to come to you by chance, you can go and look for it! If you live in or visit a suitable place, this is a very good and powerful thing to do. It's a good opportunity, too, to "switch on" and exercise the subtle awareness of the natural forces which you have been cultivating. This is an excellent project for a vacation.

Good places to look are beside water, or where water has been. The sea shore, the edges of a lake or river — particularly after a spell of dry weather when the water has receded more than usual — and, above all, completely dried out watercourses or those sandstone regions which may not have been covered with water for long ages.

Preparing for the Search

Two traditional modes of preparing yourself to seek your talisman certainly make sense. One is, to fast during the previous day. The other is, to sleep in the open at least the night previous to your quest but for more nights if you can do it. If you make this a project during a camping vacation, there's no problem.

Something more will be said about fasting in Appendix A. Meanwhile, there's this to be said in favor of it in the present context: if our primitive ancestors had nothing to eat for twenty-four hours and they then went out to look around, all their physical senses would be very sharp because, consciously or not, they'd be looking for food. To fast before this quest is probably to give yourself the advantages of that primitive sharpening of the senses.

In addition, time spent in the open air, and sleeping in the open particularly, certainly sharpens the psychic perceptions. If anyone wants an intensive course in awakening their psychic faculties, let him or her sleep in the open for a week or at least for three nights: in the back porch, in the yard, on the roof of a shed or of the house, but in nothing more than a tent and less if possible. Perhaps the psyche gets a chance to realize the physical body to which it is attached is not, after all, the only bit of "natural environment" accessible to it. However it works, fasting and sleeping out make a great combination for sharpening the physical and psychic faculties.

Your "Treasure Trove"

After that, there isn't much you can be told except simply to "go and look". (By the way, if you have fasted the day before it's a good thing to take some provisions with you on your quest. You are not here seeking for visions, simply for your talisman.)

You may pick up several objects which attract or interest you. You may, as people would in some parts of Africa, pick up a rock simply because you stub your toe on it and it seems to be trying to attract your attention that way. Gather them all. If possible, put them at this stage in separate pockets or packages. You don't want to mix them because you have not tried out their influences yet; you haven't yet adopted them into your "family".

Bring them home and live with them. You can, if need be, wash them in plain water, but do nothing else to them. From time to time, hold each one separately in your hands, place it between your palms, turn it about, "talk" to it and give it a chance to "talk" to you. If after a few days you feel there are some you want to take out again and lose them, do just that. You may end up with a few, or one you'll know is "right" for you. You could even end up with none and decide to try again another time. In that case don't be discouraged. Or the testing period may take longer than a few days. That's fine too — rocks don't eat anything.

A well-chosen Nature Talisman is an ally whose power will increase with your longer and closer association.

Charging your Talisman

You may decide you want to keep one of your rocks just as it is, while another you want to charge for a particular purpose, to have it specialize, so to put it, in focusing influences of a particular kind. You certainly don't have to charge every one of your rocks.

Supposing for instance you've collected a rock which appeals strongly to you, and which is distinctly green in color. You may feel green is a special color of yours, and the rock, just as it is, is altogether "yours". Or you may feel the green color is not so much in harmony with your personality as a good indicator for a Venus talisman, to help you to qualities you may feel you lack. Then, certainly, charge your talisman for the planetary power of Venus, according to the method given in the earlier chapters. It will not make a powerful Venusian love talisman, but it will help you gain for yourself the qualities listed under *Venus* in the final section of Chapter 4.

In other words — *if the talisman expresses qualities you feel are yours already, though maybe you'd like them strengthened, leave it as it is. If it expresses a quality you don't have but which you desire, then charge it for the appropriate planetary power for that quality.*

Setting Your Own Bounds

Many other aspects must be left aside in this general consideration of the Earth powers: the effects upon the general currents of ravines, veins of ore, hidden caves, subterranean waters. At present these subjects are truly "without end", because they are still being extensively researched. One more aspect of the matter must, however, be touched upon because it involves a practical work you can do for yourself.

You too can be the inaugurator of an area of influence among the many currents of Earth, effectively shutting out powers which might interfere with what you plan to do. Don't rush — this does not mean the time has arrived when you can enjoy the hazardous delights of making love in your own do-it-yourself zero-gravity forcefield. It does mean that many more subtle types of influence can be shut out in this way, astral influences and some which are on the borderline between the astral and the material worlds. Which is a lot simpler than delving into the researches to try to find which ones would in reality be obstructive.

The fact that you can set up barriers of this kind is in no way surprising. Minerals — whether mountain ranges or tiny samples — have their radiations, magnetic influences, lines and zones of force, as much experience testifies and as Kirlian photography confirms. Much of your body, in fact all of it in the ultimate analysis, is of the mineral world. Plants — and again experience is endorsed by Kirlian photography — radiate the power of their life-energies, set up their own resistances and barriers, and the cell-life of your body is at much the same level as that of plants. Likewise human life can parallel in itself both the rich emotional—instinctual life of the animal world, and the intellect and will whose powers are shared by non-corporeal beings. *Naturally* we can set up our own force-fields and barriers, not only spontaneously by the mere acts of existing and living, but also voluntarily and of set purpose.

The simplest way, and one of time-honored and proven effectiveness, to keep external influences from interfering with any mental or psychic work you mean to do, is that of *setting up a circle.* Besides keeping other energies out, it has also the effect of keeping your energies in, and that can be just as important.

The Circle of Power

The circle can be established in several different ways. In our book on *Psychic Self-Defense and Well-Being,* already referred to, we give several methods including the strengthening of one's personal aura by the "Tower of Light" procedure, and also the "Wall of Light" method which is most effective when performed by a number of people together. But it's good to have a variety of different defenses for different purposes, and this that will be given now is expressly intended so one person alone can powerfully set apart a larger area than just the immediate spot where he or she stands. (It can likewise be done by two people, or by several friends together, but its chief traditional use is by the power of *one* person.)

That area might be the "place of working" where you will do a charging.It might be your place of meditation. It might be your bed, or your bedroom. It might be the place where you study. It can be indoors or out. These examples will probably be enough to suggest to you the way you personally want to use the method which follows.

It is done by what is known as *"treading the circle"*.

It may not in fact be a circle. If you are short of space it can be an ellipse, or even a square or a rectangle if you want to enclose an entire room. But, if space allows, the exact circle is best to use because then your defenses will also have the strength of that perfect and outward-thrusting shape. (A hollow tube or cylinder of perfectly circular cross-section is much more difficult to bend than a solid bar of the same material and the same external dimensions. That is simply due to the uniform outward thrust and resistance of the lines of force in the circular cross-section of the cylinder.)

How long will your circular "fortress" last? If you tread it with real power, as you easily should if you've been adopting and using the various practices already given in this book, a circle established *only once* will be discernable to a perceptive dowser for at least a considerable time to come, and thus will be equally real to many other invisible influences both sentient and otherwise.

If you want to "set apart" a certain area lastingly for special purposes, you can do so by means of a simple rite.* The "treading of the circle" by itself, however, is generally supposed to last *in its full power* only until the next sunrise or

---

*So long as you keep it truly simple, and mean what you do, you can hardly go wrong with this. Having previously traced out the line of your circle, stand for a while to bring down the Light to your Heart Center, then go round the circle clockwise, sending forth the light (for this purpose) through the forefinger of your stronger hand: touching or nearly touching the ground, and visualize the traced line as shining white. Join up your circle carefully and neatly. Next, standing, you can go round the circle again, tracing at East, South, West and North whatever sign (cross, pentagram or other) most means "protection" to you. At making each sign, say something like "Be this place blessed for the works of Light, and be all harmful powers shut out from it" — or whatever formula is most meaningful to you. If you have no special Sign of Protection, trace at about eye level in the air above the first circle, another ring of white light *but this time going counter-clockwise*. This makes a traditional and potent "double lock"."

Should you feel you want for some special reason to purify the area before making the circle, first charge water: either for Saturn-Capricorn as representing the Supernal Mother governing the Earth, or for SunLeo as representing the victorious Sun purifying the "central heart" of your inner work. Prior to charging the water you can if you wish add a little natural salt (pure sea-salt or "aquarium salt"), a great cleansing and healing agent at material and astral levels. Having charged the water, sprinkle it freely about the area which is to be set apart.

This circle should not need renewing.

sunset, whichever comes first, so if you prefer the simple treading, it should be renewed every time you use the circle. To save yourself the time and trouble of repeatedly marking off your circle, you might be able to put down a circular rug you can walk around — one made of woven rushes or straw is specially harmonious for a mediation place — or you might even keep for those occasions something such as a piece of canvas with the circle marked out on it.

The Treading

Always, before beginning, fill yourself with the Light of your Higher Self.

After that, a traditional way to proceed is tread carefully around your traced circle, bringing each foot in turn to the fore and placing its heel just at the toe of the other foot. This means that every bit of the traced circular line will be really "trodden" by the sole of one of your feet in the course of your circuit. This is very thorough, very literal, and is invariable for whatever purpose you want your circle on any given occasion. It may need practice, too, to keep your balance.

Or you may feel it's more important to carry the *spirit* of your present purpose around the circle, than to create an unbroken line of footprints. This may have the good effect of bringing your inner sense of purpose to a higher level of enthusiasm, and remember, *it isn't your rational consciousness which is creative in the work of your psyche, it's your emotional-instinctual self and above all your Deep Mind.* So why not indulge your Deep Mind in its desire for freedom, for drama and play, and heighten the flow of your personal dynamism accordingly?

If your purpose on a given occasion is in harmony with one of the planetary powers — and most possible purposes are — why not pace according to the nature of that power? Never mind about the heel-to-toe business, you might go around your circle the planetary number of times, and even for Saturn and Jupiter you won't miss much of the line. (For numbers, see the Planetary Table in the course of Chapter 4.) Put on taped music, if you like. You might go with a slow, rather heavy tread for Saturn, and in a dignified and royal manner for Jupiter (but not forgetting that "joviality" requires a happy countenance). Mars can of course have a brisk *march*, but if you feel that's too obvious and easy, why not do one of those acrobatic, leaping dances which characterised the priests of Mars in ancient Rome?

For the Sun, you might while making each of your six circuits trace with your hand each of the twelve zodiacal signs in turn, or you could mime the actions of sailing in a boat (Egypt) or of driving a chariot (Greece). For Venus, a graceful light-hearted movement, full of the joy of life, is in order: cymbals, castanets, maracas, tambourine, any light percussive dance instrument is in keeping. In Ephesus (the Ephesus of the Great Mother) they shook seed pods.

And finally, for the Moon, your progress should be whatever best suits your mood. It can be fantastic and capricious, it can be dreamy and sensuous. Or, if it accords with your purpose, dreamy and sensual.

Chapter Seven

YOUNG MEN AND MAIDENS

Young men and maidens, heed my words extremely
While of the Seven Joys I tell the rhyme:
In all good faith I swear, sweet gifts and seemly
Has Love for those who render him their time.
I sing to all, but this to you supremely
Who kind and tender are and in your prime:
Know well these joys, for they are gracious things
Which Love to you, more than to others, brings.
                   Lorenzo de' Medici, "The Seven Joys of Love",
                                   transl. by Melita Denning

Because we associate radiant fitness with the image of
youthful adulthood, and of *young* adulthood above all, and
because radiant fitness is health and life in abundance,
health and life in overflowing plenty, we naturally and
rightly associate it also with sexual love.

People try to make rules about the meanings of
words, and then find themselves inarticulate in a taboo of
their own creating. The term just used must therefore be to
some extent defined: "sexual love" is intended to mean
just what it says. The word "love" does not in this context mean something which will *necessarily* hold the

117

forefront of either partner's consciousness — or even their distinct recollection — for a lifetime, but neither does it mean hate or indifference. It means the natural impulse of attraction, goodwill and heightened awareness in which one holds a fellow-being who is sharing, or who hopefully will share, a special kind of physical and emotional-instinctual delight with the lover.

It is not necessarily the same thing, either, as "falling in love", a phenomenon which certainly has a strong sexual component but which has a stronger, even a compulsive psychic element of "fascination". It is because of the dominance of the psyche in the process that people are so mistaken when they say children can't "fall in love". It is what they are very well able to do, as also are nonagenarians and many other people in whom the psyche is for whatever reason stronger than the body. Of course falling in love can and does also happen to the physically robust and fit, particularly if an apparently straightforward sexual affair develops unforseen obstacles.

"The Course of True Love . . ."

In such a case, if the obstacles don't simply put the lover off completely, they will bring the imagination into play, and once the imagination takes over, the "falling in love" situation is made. It has been said "the course of true love never did run smooth", but if it had run smooth, the true love in many instances would never have blossomed.

There is another and more mystical kind of falling in love which must be mentioned. That is the kind in which the principal "obstacle", and sometimes the only one, is engendered by a profound sense of the other's *otherness*: a glimpse of the Divine within the person. This can work out in several ways. It can console the victim of "unrequited love" with the realization that the Higher Selves of all of us exist in a bond of perfect love in the Divine Mind, or it can bring the perilous joy of the Impossible Dream into an otherwise fulfilled relationship: as the poet Coventry Patmore wrote of his wife after a number of years of happy marriage, "She's not, and never can be, mine!"

The Enjoyable Antidote

For many people, women and men alike, "falling in love" in its more intense forms is seen as something to be avoided, a distorter of sound judgment and a disorganizer of a well-planned life. One trusts to have outgrown the virulent adolescent varieties, and one hopes fervently to defer as long as possible — and perhaps to outmaneuver completely — the purple passions of later life.

People who view the matter in this way generally have no intention of living like ascetic hermits. First, they have no motivation to do any such thing. And, second, it usually doesn't work. If a person seriously wants to be an ascetic hermit, they need to find a place and a mode of life in which to be it thoroughly, besides having some good permanent motivation. But to try to avoid the more drastic forms of fascination by shutting sexual love out of your life entirely, is in most cases to build up the sort of inner "obstacle" mentioned just above, which can work somewhat like an electrical resistance, building up the current to a force which unexpectedly kicks you right into the very thing you were trying to keep away from.

That may be your personal view of the matter, or it may not. Certainly, with regard to life's other stresses and crises, sex is an excellent *re-creation*, an unbuilding and rebuilding of the partners, and usually a resultant restoration of things to a plainer and saner perspective.

What Sex Isn't

At least, sex should be that kind of haven, that kind of *play*. To make it so, you may need to realize — or to help your partner realize — that sex itself isn't just one more thing to get stressed up about. It's happy, it's fun!

Some learned theories are going around these days about the right way to have sex, about standards of performance and so on. If those things bother either of you, forget them. You don't have sex with your intellect. Sex isn't a competition in performance. It is not a test in orgasmic ability. It is not a school of any kind. Neither (with or without marriage) is it an activity which gives any religious or other person or institution a right to ask how, when, where or why you make love (as if you were minors or insane.) In the relationship between you and your lover, no opinions matter except those of the two of you. If you have a good relationship, enjoy it.

The Way You Look

Success in sexual relationships has little to do with standard ideas about beauty or good looks, either. Women, as a fact, seem to realize this more easily than men. Once it gets through to a woman that her lovers are not particularly concerned about the shape of her toes, for instance, or the fact that she may have one breast noticeably bigger than the other, she can go her ways with the air of a goddess. But if a man finds his personal appearance lacking, and particularly if he thinks his penis is not average length, or is no more than average length, he may take a lot of reassuring.

That particular male sensitivity, however, can have a positive aspect. An overweight man, or the lover of an overweight man, might consider this as an encouragement to him in the matter of losing weight. It's predictable that this can be demonstrated in front of the bathroom mirror: at least one more precious penial inch can be temporarily revealed by lifting the fatty tissue at the base of the abdomen, and, by properly dieting and exercising away that fatty tissue, can be permanently reclaimed!

Every man and every woman owe it to themselves and also to their lovers and friends, to look their fittest and best. "Beauty" is not expected, and, by itself, is not what attracts; some of the most sexually attractive men and women are, and throughout history have been, far too individual in their appearance to measure to the conventional standard of good looks, whether female or male. A body well cared for and esteemed by its owner, the sparkle of fitness, with good grooming and the poise of knowing one's own style; these are the qualities which attract not only love, but the respect which makes for the ongoing success of a relationship.

Fruits of Self-Confidence

Usually when people ask advice on how to be more popular, gain sex appeal, find a lover, they are advised to manifest qualities of sympathy, kindness, generosity, to be a good listener and so on. That sort of advice is very good in principle, but is frequently not of much use to the people it's addressed to. It can make serious problems for them, besides, by putting them psychically in a false position and causing them to fall prey to parasitic flatterers. The first thing they need is more self-confidence, more true sense of self-worth.

Consider, for comparison, the type of person you sometimes see who, no matter how well dressed, ruins the whole effect by constantly worrying about his or her attire: making sure a tie or pendant is central, fingering a collar, checking that a jacket sits right, and so on. An unthinking observer might suppose this to be a very vain, self-admiring person, whereas just the opposite is likely to be true; here is someone who is painfully stressed with doubts as to his or her whole appearance. The image suggests a total lack of self-confidence.

So it is also with the matters we are considering. The

self-confident people, the ones who radiate inner fitness, don't need telling to show generosity and sympathy. They possess, and manifest, cordiality and compassion unconsciously even — with a gleam of sexual fire — because that's the natural way for people to be, and only fear and self-doubt make them otherwise. Such people don't ask how to find friends, how to find a lover; they joyfully reach out a hand to the friend or the lover chosen, and often are just as joyfully accepted. Should it prove otherwise there may be regrets, but no occasion for any painful soul-searching.

If you are happy with yourself, you can be happy with other people and they with you. Furthermore — and this you'll need in those circumstances — you'll have the inner strength to brush off the ones you *don't* want around you.

The Earthly Paradise

If you are an enthusiast for radiant fitness, to give expression to that radiance in sexual love can have marvelous effects in stepping up the glandular and nervous tone of your body, so that your fitness becomes more radiant —more visibly radiant to all beholders — than it was before. Likewise the imaginative and creative powers of your psyche are enhanced, as, inevitably, your heightened awareness of your "significant other" adds new dimensions, new lights and shades, to the world as you individually have perceived it. It is this savoring and exploration of another personality, almost as it were from the inside, which gives an ecstatic intensity to the physical sexual experience itself, beyond the scope of any other physical pleasure to equal.

If your lover is also an enthusiast for radiant fitness, then the shared experience is more than doubled, it is (to borrow a mathematical term) lifted to another "power" altogether.

To Encourage the Men

Here a usual question needs to be answered. these heightened joys of sexual gratification: what will they do for the men? Are the male participants not going to be exhausted and enervated by their repeated losses of glandular secretions, blood sugar and essential proteins at every orgasm? Will their physical and mental energy not deteriorate rapidly?

There are several parts to the answer to this.

1. People generally (this clause refers to women as well as men) who don't cultivate radiant inner fitness, with its vital co-ordination of "healthy mind with healthy body", have little idea of their real potential for sexual pleasure.

2. *Better* sex doesn't necessarily, therefore, mean *more* sex. In many instances, and especially at first, better sex can mean fewer hours spent vainly seeking elusive satisfaction; hence better nerves, greater fitness and still more intensified sexual powers. In a "radiant fitness" twosome, the keener sensations and more expressive bodily response of each partner to the other will also greatly enhance the pleasure of both.

3. At the same time radiant fitness, continually working from the psyche through the activated and synchronized bodily structures, will certainly—given a good natural regimen of life — build up a man's potential for sexual performance to levels which the present-day artificial culture around us has largely come to regard as "legendary". In lands of central Europe, where rural living has preserved more healthful conditions, a man of notable sexuality is described as having "a good back". Those people are right. Posture, breathing and exercise all have their part to play here; besides, of course, diet, of which

more in the next chapter.

4. Seminal fluid does however represent a high concentration of valuable life-sustaining ingredients, and there is no reason for its wasteful expenditure. (Involuntary losses of an excess are of course nothing to worry about.) The question at the opening of this section is worded as it is, because that's the way most people around us still think about it. In reality, however, "orgasm" is by no means synonymous with "ejaculation". (People who make that confusion are at a loss to explain how women have orgasms, if indeed they can accept that women do.) With some practice, a number of orgasms can be enjoyed, to the progressively increasing pleasure of both partners, without ejaculation. The method for postponed or non-occurring ejaculation, derived from the traditions of Tao, is given in step-by-step detail in *The Magick of Sex.** It is a technique rapidly finding favor in the West for the enhanced well-being, intensified pleasure and potential for pleasure, and renewed joy in living, which it brings to man and woman alike.†

Widening the Perspective

If you and your lover want to keep your relationship to simple levels of physical and cultural fun, that's great in itself. Besides having sex together, it might include enjoying sports together (both active and spectator), listening to music together, going to shows, movies, whatever you both

---

Practical Guide to the Magick of Sex, by Melita Denning and Osborne Phillips (Llewellyn).

†Women who have studied the Chinese literature on the psycho-physical practices of Tao are sometimes disturbed because the exclusive concern of the writings appears to be with the benefits to the male practitioner. Both reason and the experience of many couples, however, indicate equal, if not greater, benefits for the female. It must be remembered that in old-time China the women practitioners of Tao were an elite of intelligent and highly trained professionals. They were offering a service to the men: it would have been in no way to their advantage to publicize the benefits to themselves also.

like. If it includes hiking, biking or boating together, that's a wonderful booster for the radiant fitness of both of you at every level! None of these things need make for too intense a commitment, but they do give you and your lover a chance for that exploration into each other's personalities, each other's special ways of viewing and doing things, which is one of the most important psychic aspects, and one of the most permanently enriching experiences, of any relationship.

If one or the other of you has a motive for keeping your affair a secret — which in any case is sensible if you work at the same place, only do arrange things so it won't be the end of the world if the secrecy breaks down — this will impair your chances for shared activity. All the more reason, in those circumstances, to find an opportunity now and again for time together out in the country or on the water, to break the tension.

Exploring More Deeply

It's splendid, however, if both of you feel you would like your shared relationship to include some exploration of those inner levels of the psyche of which you both individually will have gained a more conscious awareness through your practices for radiant fitness.

You can build up the interaction of your two Deep Minds in a number of fun ways. Here are a few games you and your lover can play at odd moments: remember to keep them as "games" — almost childish games — and you'll do far better than if you take them too seriously. In matters you take seriously, the rational consciousness will step in and try to take a hand — and the rational consciousness just can't do this sort of thing.

1. *Telepathy and Visualization*   You need a plain surface of about 12 by 12 inches; it could well be larger. A dark surface is best: a small chalkboard, the back of a photo album or a

large-format book in a dark binding, anything fairly large and plain. One of you holds it up almost vertically — perhaps with the edge resting on the knees — so as to be able to gaze at it comfortably, and so the other partner can also look at it from the side or over the shoulder. (It is better if the second partner does not watch the board at first.) The person with the board gazes at it, and imagines, drawn upon it as if in chalk and fairly large, a geometric figure in outline: a circle, triangle, square, five- or six-pointed star, anything which is not too complex to visualize easily and which the other person is likely to be able to name. Then the other person is asked what it is.

That person may get the name by simple telepathy, but when you both have some practice it should be no problem for each partner to "see", as if physically, the white outline the other has projected upon the board.

2. *Card Guessing* This can be played with ESP cards if you happen to have them — they are so very clear and distinct — but if not, ordinary playing cards will do. There are two versions; the first is termed "cards seen". One partner takes a deck of cards, well shuffled to avoid getting a run of one suit, and, holding them so the other can't see the faces of the cards, looks at the first one. The other partner has to name the card being looked at, either instantaneously, or after a moment's reflection, at choice. You may find it interesting, if you use playing cards, to see whether each of you scores right more often with the number or with the suit; this may depend on both the "sender" and the "receiver".

After some practice with this, you may care to try a much more mysterious form of the game, which must depend simply upon the powers of the Deep Mind. Nevertheless, some people are remarkably good at it. It is termed "cards unseen".

After shuffling, the deck is laid face down upon the table. The top card is removed carefully and is laid, still face down, a little distance from the deck. Each partner writes down what card he or she thinks it is. The next card is now carefully removed from the deck and is laid, still face down, on top of the first card, and each partner writes down what he or she thinks it is. And so on, for as many cards as the two of you want to try.

Then you turn over the newly stacked cards, and compare them with your lists. One of the interesting things, of course, is to see how many each of you got right, but more interesting is to see how far you both got *the same ones* right. And when you got them wrong, did the two of you make the same wrong "guess"?

3. *"Hot Trail"* This is a simple version of a game which was devised for a number of people; initially, in fact, for a whole family named Murray. One of you being out of the room, the other one touches, or just fixedly looks at, a particular object. (Going out of the room is practically essential, as a person with sharp ears has no difficulty in hearing, quite often, even someone's head turn to look at something!) The "banished" one then returns and has to discover the object. Again, this may be done simply by telepathy, but the seeker is entitled to go about the room touching things with the fingertips, or holding the center of the palm slightly above them. The game gets its name from the slight sensation of warmth often felt in the object that has been touched or even simply looked at.

You may find that the two of you are alike in some things, but sharply contrasted in others. While no very profound significance should be read into these matters, they all help you both explore what kind of relationship you have, out of the infinite number of "mix and match" varieties.

Should you want to delve more deeply into matters of ESP, scrying, psychometry and so on, it's all open to you. That is where our book on *The Development of Psychic Powers* previously referred to could be of further help to you. For the present, however, the emphasis here is on your relationship as lovers.

There's Magick and . . .

There's a neat little piece of magick the two of you can do together, if you'd care to try your powers. Some people don't like the word "magick", but what is wanted is a word to mean "the psychic power to make things happen" which is a little more general in its use than such terms as psychokinesis, hypnosis, psychic healing, which of course are all psychic ways of making things happen. The thing which will be described for you is really a special form of creative visualization; only creative visualization in itself is usually done by one person alone and without using any added energy source.

Usually it can be said that the kinds of magick which people find off-putting or scary are those which they see as unaccountable, irrational. Although doing something irrational — such as singing a nonsense rhyme — can truly be helpful in allowing our powerful Deep Mind to get into action instead of our less powerful rational mind, people often need to get used to this.

In the procedure to be given here, nothing needs to be done which you have not already encountered, and had explained, in this book.

A Simple Piece of Sex Magick

This is one of the simplest kinds of sex magick two people can perform, but it can be very effective.

First, choose a night for it: a night when you mean to make love, and if practicable, a night of the Full Moon. Otherwise, choose a time when the moon is increasing. Be sure to avoid the waning moon for this, because — as people have always realized — the moon is of great power and importance in all matters concerned with love and sex.

To begin with, it's good if one of you will charge some water for the Moon — simply the "planetary" power, no zodiacal sign — and the other one will lightly sprinkle this on and about the bed or whatever place you have decided upon for your lovemaking. (Of course people don't always choose a bed — it might be a rug or a cupped hilltop or a reedbrake or anywhere else; but from now, for convenience, we'll call it "the bed".) Next you both should perform the nine rounds of the bed, pacing or dancing — even running if you wish, taking turns to catch up with each other; that would accord well with what you are doing, but keep count of the nine circuits — and sealing finally with the four signs or the reverse circle. You can both do the signs if you wish, but it should be done back to back; that is to say, if you sign East, South, West, North, your lover should at the same time sign West, North, East, South, and if you move counter-clockwise East, North, West, South, your lover should keep pace with you while moving West, South, East, North. This is easier to do than to read or write, but in all cases both of you should take care to move on, after completing your circle, to that next point which you started from.

The action, from this point on, is the way the two of you want it. *But you should each of you manage, as long as this love session continues, to call to mind as often and as vividly as you can, some special thing you desire.* Preferably it should be some special thing you've agreed between you beforehand, or you can each have your own separate objective; but the agreed, shared objective is usually by far the more potent. Neither of you should just "wish" for whatever your objective may be: visualize it, even before you enter the circle. Then, as you proceed with your lovemaking, "see" it becoming energized, almost materialized, by the sexual energy given off by yourself and your lover, *which is kept from dispersing by the ninefold Moon-circle you have created round about.*

With this incentive, you will want on this occasion particularly to build up that energy as high as you can. There are two things you can do to make sure of this, other than (or besides, if it suits your plans) having a little feast of aphrodisiac — desire-making — foods and drinks beforehand.* The first good thing in your lovemaking, on this type of occasion especially, is to build up as intense a current as possible in and between the two of you, by means of the most skillfully prolonged "powerhousing" — mutual stimulation with hand and mouth — you can both endure. (If you are both into the Tao technique mentioned earlier in this chapter, that's an excellent variant here too). *But don't forget to return your attention to your visualization between whiles, building the energy into it with your will.* The second important point is, when you come to the definitive coitus for the grand climax of the session, really to let yourselves go. The moment of entry (on that occasion, in case you have had preparatory ones in accord with the Tao practice)

---

*Usually, for two people actively pursuing radiant fitness, such a procedure is neither necessary nor desirable. The healthy body, left to make its own pace, will produce in the bloom of fitness enough superabundance of energy for a full and happy sex life. A special occasion now and then, however, is another matter. Some alcoholic drinks in moderation can be good, but each person has to know his or her limits and idiosyncracies to avoid defeating the intended purpose. For food, the non meat eater has eggs, normal mushrooms and of course an interesting range of botanicals. (it should be noted that the effect on vegetarians of alcohol and any drugs — including ordinary cooking spices, and tobacco — is relatively greater than on meat eaters.) Those vegetable substances which are reputed to have aphrodisiac qualities, but which are also hallucinogens, may attract some people to try them — *with a prior good understanding of their properties* — when the object is pleasure simply. I, the author, do not make that recommendation being of the opinion that (a) sex is usually better enjoyed "with a clean palate", and (b) that in the present context particularly, the "clouding" effect can be detrimental to the full force of creative will.

Meat eaters have other options besides the above: raw oysters are traditional, and there is a very notable modern Roman dish (its properties merit for it to have been Imperial Roman too) of beef braised with red wine and other ingredients.

should be, for both partners, the signal for the great affirmation of *the achieved reality* of the visualized objective. At that moment — not before — bring down the Light of your Higher Self into the visualized image to "lock" it. If you and your lover are visualizing the same thing, you should both conceive here that you are each bringing down the Light of your own Higher Self into *the one shared image*, giving it "life".* Don't doubt! It is an accepted fact among people who are familiar with these things — all the world over — that this technique *works*. "See" it as an accomplished fact. After that, if either of you can cling to, or revert to, that realization, do so up to the final orgasm. In the nature of things, there are likely to be several orgasms from that final entry until the end. Neither of you should spare anything, either in body language or vocally, to make the emotional-instinctual release on this occasion as total as possible.

Then — it hardly needs saying — simply let all visualizations naturally fade. The physical and psychic levels of both of you will quietly reabsorb any unused energies which may remain, including those of the circle itself.

---

*If the desired objective is not an easily visualized material object, the best procedure here (differently from that required for the Sex Magick technique given in *The Magick of Sex*) is to visualize *a person* having the desired quality. The person visualized should be of the same sex as the intended recipient, unless it is a quality you both desire; then it should be a young child of indeterminate sex. If you both want to qualify as doctors, for instance, "see" the child as destined for that profession. But if a specific sum of money is needed, there is no better course than to visualize it — perhaps in a bank account, or written on a check — but be sure to name and to visualize the amount in figures.

Chapter Eight

SOME HAE MEAT . . .

Some hae meat an' canna eat,
Some hae nane that want it:
But we hae meat an' we can eat,
An' sae the Lord be thankit!
Traditional Scots Grace before Meals

Out civilization today presents us with a curious paradox. Poverty in the world, and the suffering caused by poverty, are grievous but cannot astonish us. These are, and have long been, familiar evils. What is only now coming to public attention is the amount of suffering, and indeed of grave sickness, due to improper diet and inadequate ways of living, which afflicts the people of prosperous countries.

Plainly then, prosperity in itself is not the complete answer. As King Midas discovered in the legends of this same civilization's childhood, you can't eat money — not even in its most attractive form, bullion — not even if you spend twenty-four hours a day acquiring it. People can be well dressed, well shod, well housed, with plenty of money for extras, and yet be inadequately nourished.

One meets numberless people who complain that if

they are to get through a day's work they can't spare the energy to exercise; so they eat more food to get more energy. Then, however, they put on excess weight and have even less energy for exercise, because of the effort needed to lift those surplus pounds around.

Until very lately, it has been the fashion to blame this state of affairs entirely on the quality of the available foodstuffs. That is a part of the answer, but only a part. It is now coming to public realization also, that the food we eat is not our only source of energy. Nevertheless, let's look at the food question first.

Heaven knows, there's no shortage of food in the world, although there are appalling problems in its distribution. Part of the problem which concerns us here is neither the quantity nor, initially, the quality of foodstuffs produced for people in our society, but the ruin and denaturization of many of those foodstuffs before they reach the public.

Tackling Our Food Problem

In this as in other things, it's no use expecting the scene to be changed until it changes from within, and that has to be a result of each person's actions. This means a certain amount of trouble-taking and perhaps of inconvenience in the early stages, but for more fitness, more enjoyment of life, isn't it worth it?

The busy shopper may know of the perniciousness of fine-ground flour and the "inflated" loaf, for instance, but very likely the small local store sells no other type of bread. There may be a healthier selection at the supermarket (which may be crowded) or you may do better still at a health food store if you know of one and if they aren't too expensive.

With regard to bread particularly, there is something of a difficulty. Not only may the good whole grain loaf be really rather more expensive, pound for pound, than the popular loaf, but, to the eye accustomed to the "inflated" type of bread, it looks much smaller. Frequently people don't read the weight on the label, they only look at the *volume* of what they are buying. It takes the experience of good bread to discover how much less of it, in volume, you need to be well satisfied at a meal. It even happens that the mother of a family may make it an *objection* that her children eat fewer slices of the good bread, while in fact it is giving them much better nourishment.*

(Incidentally, on the subject of inducing more people to do some of their grocery shopping at health food stores, it would help if the staff at some health food stores could bring themselves to look as if they were selling the kinds of food a normal person should be eating — which is for the most part the truth of the matter — instead of having that air of being dedicated attendants at some kind of shrine, ministering only to the needs of the Illuminated. It scares newcomers.)

Happily, more and more supermarkets are beginning to realize that there is an aware and growing public for unprocessed or minimally processed foods, and to provide them accordingly. Some have a special "health" section, others simply display those foods among the rest under their appropriate classification. If you read the labels and shop carefully, you may not come out with an overloaded cart, but you will have food which you can eat with an assurance of nourishment yourself, or give with a clear conscience to anyone else you may be shopping for. Increased sales of the better quality foods will encourage increased production of them, and this should mean a reduction of

---

*NOTE: If bread is labeled "whole wheat", wheat and wheat alone provides its flour content. But you don't get the whole wheat grain, including the germ, unless the bread is labeled "whole grain" and "stone ground". You can't. Without the slower speed of stone grinding, the wheat germ if included would literally "gum up the works".

their prices to at least the same level as "junk non-food". (Increased demand doesn't by any means always send prices up. If manufacturers know they can count on a large number of consumers for a product, naturally the setting up and staffing of its production can be costed out at a lower rate per consumer than if only a minority market is anticipated.) It will take time to achieve this goal, but meanwhile in any case you'll be living better.

Some Miscellaneous Food Pointers

The authors of the classic cookbook, *Joy of Cooking,* say in their introductory article on *The Foods We Eat,* "Nutrition is concerned not with food as such, but with the substances that food contains." True: but unfortunately we can't reverse the statement. The substances that food contains are sometimes hardly remotely concerned with nutrition.

As a general rule, go for the label which indicates the fewest additives. "Enriching" is a thing you have to do your thinking about. If milk has been pasteurized and is subsequently "enriched" with vitamins, that's fine and probably puts the milk back where it ought to be. Louis Pasteur found out about "bugs" and how to kill them, but he knew nothing about vitamins and so couldn't realize that you kill them just the same way. An enriched loaf of bread is another matter. Sometimes lightweight bread is enriched so that slice for slice it contains about the same nutrients as a good loaf. But it's still lightweight: therefore you and anyone else you are shopping for will still eat six slices of it instead of two, so that for dietetic purposes you've eaten about a quarter of a loaf and probably are still hungry.

Nobody, but nobody of any age, needs commercially produced cookies, cakes, or candies or salted crackers. The flour (when they have it) is wrong, the fat is wrong, the sugar is wrong, the synthetic colorings and flavorings and the preservatives are wrong. No matter whether you need to lose weight or not, avoid those things and stay with fresh fruit to nibble on, if nibble you must. Or unsalted sunflower or melon seeds. As for temptation, if you never buy the junk things you'll never find them in your refrigerator and your cupboard.

If you have children to cater for, don't weaken! Apart from the pitfall for the adults, you should avoid conditioning the children with a taste which may make problems for them all their days. Give them better things in life, let them share outdoor fun and adventure with you, and they won't rate you a spoilsport but will respect your opinions.

Mix your own breakfast cereal. Natural rolled oats are a good basis, but if you feel your digestion or your teeth might not be up to that, *Quaker Oats* gives you two other choices: the "old fashioned", which is quite a lot softer than the natural article, and the almost melt-in-your-mouth "Quick Quaker". You can buy either of those two last products very economically in 42-ounce packs. Put a handful in a bowl and add a tablespoonful each of other items. You might choose raw wheat germ, millet flakes, unsalted sunflower seeds, even a pure processed grain like one of *Kellogg's Nutri-Grain* range, or *Grape Nuts*. Or, if you have *Shredded Wheat*, you could use in your mix all those little broken bits which collect in the bottom of the pack.

You can add more recondite items, too, to benefit yourself in particular ways: a spoonful of lecithin granules perhaps, and/or a spoonful of brewers yeast.

Mix all your dry ingredients well together before adding the milk. If you are using skim milk to cut down on fats, here's how you can obtain a nice creamy consistency and do yourself some extra good besides: Get some skim milk *powder* and mix a spoonful in with your other dry ingredients. Then add your liquid milk. That way, you avoid the fat and have double the valuable milk-minerals instead.*

A mix of this type is delicious in itself, but if you feel you must have some kind of sweetener, use a little honey or blackstrap molasses, or add fruit.

About Fruit Drinks

With milk, which is a food, and your daily quota of water, you need never consider any other cold drink except pure fruit juices. You may buy them concentrated and frozen, or reconstituted and ready to use — both these are completely acceptable — but don't buy anything which describes itself as a "drink": whether apple drink, orange juice drink, grape juice drink or other. Or "orangeade." On examination, you'll find that the percentage of the genuine juice is usually around 9% or even lower. The substances sold as this or that *flavor* can, of course, be completely synthetic.

None of them are worth considering. Keep with the real thing. Generally speaking you are not planning to live on fruit juice, and if for a short time you are (see Appendix A, on Fasting) you'll do better to buy the fruit itself.

All the fruit juices are good and healthful drinks, rich in vitamins and minerals which will benefit you in various ways. Sometimes choose one, sometimes another to get the good of all. For a cold drink in hot weather, however, choose tomato. It's the one fruit juice which contains less natural sugar even than lemon, and so for keeping you feeling cool, relaxed and unsticky it has no equal.

A splendid fruit juice whose properties have been much controverted, is grapefruit. Many people discovered in the sixties that grapefruit (fruit or juice) is excellent for

---

*If you want to step up your system's power of absorbing from your food the calcium you need for good bones and teeth, make a habit of concluding your main meal with a small glass of fruit juice. Apple juice is excellent for this purpose.

trimming and toning the figure. Unfortunately the people who were helped by it, and recommended it to others, mostly couldn't say *why* it worked, and the critics who derided it likewise did so with no understanding of the matter.

So let's say at once, okay, grapefruit has calories. Grapefruit contains sugar, although less sugar than, for instance, an orange. Grapefruit contains "fat" — the aromatic oil which makes it smell like grapefruit. But the loss of fatty tissue — which is the most important objective in weight loss — involves some vital factors besides calories, fats and sugars.

One of the problems is water trapped in the tissues. Alcohol makes this problem worse, because alcohol, wherever found — and it does get into the body tissues of these who drink it — will attract and hold water. Another thing that makes it worse is the quantity of pollutants in modern food, which the system has never evolved adequate means of throwing off; they might be flushed out by the circulation, but instead they tend to get trapped in these "sandbanks" of waterlogged fatty tissue. Just as blackheads cause enlarged pores on the outer skin, so these unwholesome deposits distend the inner tissues and cause "flab".

To combat that situation, a person needs (1) exercise, not only to tone the muscles but to step up the circulation. Talk about exercise "turning fat into muscle" is nonsense: fat is fat and muscle is muscle. But muscle can increase the circulation and it can also, so to speak, "massage" the fat from the inside; (2) plenty of water, so that the system *can* be cleared, and also because water carries purifying and activating oxygen; and (3) something to speed the water, with the impurities it has gathered, out of the system: that is, a *diuretic*.

Grapefruit juice is a diuretic. For the best results, a small glass of it — the usual kind of small juice glass, about 2/3 of a cup or five ounces — should be drunk first thing every morning, before any other drink or food. As a regular practice, this is an excellent promoter of those clean, firm contours which, in this present decade, are coming to be recognized as one of the most desired signs of radiant fitness in man and woman alike.

It confers another benefit as well. Taken that way, as the first thing swallowed in the morning, its fresh, unsweet flavor provides a good "education" for the taste buds. It's a fact that the less they are pampered with sweet flavors, the less they will crave such. Grapefruit juice "sets the tone" in every way.

Citrus Allergy?

For people who unfortunately can't use grapefruit because of a citrus allergy, a very good healthful cold drink to take on arising is a blend of raw vegetable juices. Such blends can be bought bottled or canned. Vegetable juices are excellent blood purifiers and promoters of radiant fitness in their own ways, and these drinks likewise give you that clean, unsweet start to the day.

Something Preservatives Don't Preserve

You probably have realized that most of the yogurt offered for sale, besides being sweetened, is inert and worthless apart from some vitamins which may remain in the fruit that's mixed with it. You may therefore decide to include in your diet only really natural and unsweetened yogurt — labeled "Natural" and not just "Natural Flavor" — a noble food which has been a staple article of diet for a number of people in Turkey and eastward from there, who've kept most of their faculties to a hale 120 years and over.

Okay, you track down a supply of this authentic yogurt, and you'd like some fruit with it. *Be sure to use fresh fruit for this purpose, raw or stewed! Don't even use dried fruit.* The reason is this. In keeping fruit, one of the chief problems is to avoid the development of a yeast culture. (Which is why wine, good or bad, can be made from most any kind of fruit. The ferment which produces the wine is set up by a yeast.) So when bottled fruit, fruit conserve, jam, jelly or syrup, contains a preservative, you can be sure this preservative will be chosen precisely to destroy yeasts. But some yeasts are extremely beneficial to you, and the ferment which gives your genuine natural yogurt its high food value is one of these yeasts, and if you mix it with preserved fruit, you kill it dead.

Incidentally, what is technically known as the "flora" in your intestinal tract is also a type of yeast very much like the one in the yogurt. So if you were to make a *habit* of eating jellies, preserves and dried fruit instead of fresh raw or stewed fruit, you could be depriving yourself of that beneficial population as well.

Vegetables: Cooked or Raw?

Most vegetables, both green and root, are, on balance, best eaten raw. (Only don't make a coleslaw an excuse for an orgy of mayonnaise dressing!) Certainly they have a considerably higher calorie count when raw, but this is more than compensated — for most people — by the higher vitamin content and by the fact that they are more satisfying. A fair-sized carrot, for instance, grated raw, is a very acceptable vegetable to accompany most things you might eat cooked carrot with, but you might easily eat twice as much cooked carrot.

The one exception to this recommendation of raw vegetables is the potato, whether sweet or Irish. (No one, I suppose, is going to attempt eating a raw yam!) There has been a kind of fad among health-food enthusiasts of recent years, for eating Irish potatoes sliced, raw or nearly raw. This is *not* a healthy practice. The Irish potato is acceptable as an article of human diet only on certain terms: you should eat only those tubers which are completely sound and mature, and they should be thoroughly well cooked. The best of all ways to cook them is to bake them in their jackets. The next best is to scrub but not peel them, cut them up and boil them. If you stick a fork in a piece of boiled potato, the potato should break.

If you want an accompaniment to your potato but for reasons of diet want to avoid the fat content of butter or sour cream, use cottage cheese; particularly the low-fat variety. You will probably not feel you've made any sacrifice. Those low-calorie margarines are not usually a good idea. If in doubt, take up a pack or tub and read the ingredients. The foremost, or nearly the foremost, will be water: then you get an assortment of fats, emulsifiers, artificial flavorings and colors, and very often among the rest there are, after all, "milk solids" as well. So, doctor's orders excepted, you may well decide to stay with real butter and eat it more sparingly. Besides, you can have salt-free butter if you wish. (Or you could give it a miss altogether and have even fewer calories to count, but such a good nutrient should not be unthinkingly discarded.)

Low Fat Meats

If you eat meat — whether you want to lose weight, build up muscle, or just stay as trim as you are — low-fat meats should be your choice. Many books on dieting list chicken as a low-fat meat. Low-fat it is not, certainly not the disjointed chicken pieces packaged in the supermarkets. In a matter of that kind, you have to use your own eyes and do your own thinking. Lamb, a very digestible meat, is generally considered as too full of fat, and for that reason is not recommended. It is fatty, but can easily be defatted by the time-honored method of stewing, chilling overnight, and then removing the fat easily as a solid sheet from the surface of the stew. Some people do that twice, the result being as fat-free a dish as a meat eater could wish for. Fish is usually listed as low-fat, but it ought to be mentioned that this description doesn't apply to sardines, salmon or herring, in whatever way prepared. "Lean beef" — that is, beef without a noticeable amount of fat in the "grain" — with external fat trimmed off and either stewed or grilled, according to the cut, is probably among the meat-eater's best choices for general purposes. For minerals, "organ meats" are the most valuable source.

About Vegetables, Fruit, Grains

A vegetarian can, with care, live well and very healthily without meat. Simply being a vegetarian is not enough, as regards health. One might be a vegetarian and live — while one lived — on pasta and candies, or one might be like the cheerful alcoholic in G.K. Chesterton's poem:

> No more the milk of cows
> Shall pollute my private house
> Than the milk of the wild mares of the barbarian:
> But I'll feast on port and sherry
> Because I am so very,
> So very, very, very vegetarian!

Strictly, it's doubtful whether being a vegetarian on a less than well-organized diet is satisfactory on ethical grounds either, if the intention is to avoid the abuse of animals. As St. Francis of Assisi realized late in his life (he left this world at the age of forty-five), one's body is also an animal and is entitled to fair treatment.

The chief difficulty in the vegetarian diet is to get adequate protein. This is often obtained from non-vegetable sources such as eggs, milk and milk products, though the cheddars are said to be the only adequate cheeses. Among vegetable foods, nuts are excellent. The whole bean tribe, too, has for centuries been counted upon, not only by people who reckoned themselves to be vegetarians, byt by that unnumbered multitude — a great part of the population of medieval Europe — who for economic, social or ecological reasons seldom or never had any meat available to them. Several kinds of beans are in common use nowadays, but for the person who does not eat meat as well, the two most notable are the soy bean and the Lima bean.

Soy products take all kinds of forms. Lima beans are one of the few vegetables which are to be preferred frozen rather than fresh-picked. For a quick, high-protein meatless snack which is tempting enough to appeal to anyone, grate beforehand a serving of cheddar cheese. Boil or steam the frozen Lima beans, drain them quickly and dish, and heap the grated cheese over them so that it melts with the heat of the beans.

While a vegetarian can live, and live well, without meat, a meat eater certainly cannot live without vegetable foods. In the animal world, even the true carnivores will occasionally eat various herbs, grass, even fruit. The nutrients of vegetable life are indispensable. Green vegetables, and the edible seaweeds, are valuable to help purify the blood and to guard us from various ills according to their kind. Yellow vegetables — such as pumpkin, squash, carrot, sweet potatoes and yams — are good for bones, skin and eyes, and for the functioning of the digestive tract. Onions, besides containing sulphur (which in itself is a famous old "home remedy") have a pungent oil which brings them, with their even more potent relatives the garlics, high on the list of our healers and helpers. Mushrooms contain iodine and riboflavin, and broccoli contains ascorbic acid. For most people, however, the great sources of ascorbic acid are always the fruits: strawberries and the citrus fruits notably. The list could be prolonged. A varied intake of fruit and vegetables of all kinds is, in the interests of health and fitness, a good project for everyone.

What Starch Do You Favor?

Every diet includes some type of starchy food, because we need starch for energy. Such foods come from seeds such as wheat, corn and the other grains — beechnuts and acorns ("oak corn") have also been used — or from tubers and roots such as the various potatoes, and such as the manioc root which, with its poisonous juice removed, gives tapioca. Whatever may be enjoyed by way of variety, most people have one favorite, basic starch food: one of the kinds of potato, bread made from one or more grains, cornmeal, pasta made from wheat flour, beans (which are another type of seed), lentils and so on. They are a source of some protein as well as starch; but many of them are "enemies" if you are seriously tackling a weight problem!

A Healthful Basic Food

If you want a very healthful basic starch food, and particularly if you want to lose weight without losing out on energy, try brown rice. White rice is of no use. Brown rice mixes well with peas and with any of the kinds of lentil. They can be used separately for variety, but also they mix well together and their various properties balance nicely.

Peas and lentils cook easily: brown rice takes rather longer, although I have never known it to take its reputed forty minutes. Because of the cooking time, some people object to cooking it in small portions; also, while rice is cooking the pot needs to remain covered, and this makes a difficulty if rice is added in with other raw ingredients to make a stew, for instance, which needs stirring and testing from time to time. My recommendation is that you cook at one time the largest potful you can, remembering to allow for its considerable expansion. When cooked, allow it to stand for five minutes and drain off any remaining liquid (don't throw it away — drink it or put it in soup). Then, after the rice is cool, measure it by the cupful into thin sandwich-size plastic bags. Twist the top of each bag — no need to tie — and put them all in the freezer. As you will be heating each bagful when used, it's best not to cook it over-soft to begin with.

You might cook together carrot, onion and anything else you might wish for a good vegetable stew, then add the precooked brown rice, heat through, and so make it into a complete meal. Or here's a suggestion for a well balanced, and delicious, baked or grilled meal:

Spicy Vegetable Cheesebake

Thaw out, if frozen, 3 cupfuls of precooked brown rice. Cook 1 cup fresh or frozen peas. Meantime, place in a skillet (with a very small amount of vegetable oil) 2 medium carrots, thinly sliced; 2 medium onions, thinly sliced; one-half cup fresh parsley, chopped; and 1 teaspoon powdered paprika. When the onions and carrots are soft, mix in 2 cups mushrooms, peeled and sliced; 2 cloves garlic, peeled and finely chopped; and about one-half teaspoon fresh ginger, peeled and finely chopped. Saute for another 60 seconds, then add 2 teaspoons tamari or soy sauce. Salt is optional.

Strain the peas, mix these and the vegetable mixture into the 3 cups brown rice. Put the whole mixture into a lightly oiled shallow casserole or metal baking dish, then pile on top 3 cups grated cheddar cheese. If liked, a few slices of tomato can be placed on the rice and vegetable mix before topping with cheese.

Bake for 30 minutes at 350°; or, if a metal dish is used, it can be cooked under the grill until the cheese begins to brown.

Lentils again

For a rich, spicy accompaniment to other foods, cook one-half cup (measured raw) of red or brown lentils with a tablespoon of lemon juice in the water, one-half teaspoon dried sweet basil, and a pinch of powdered nutmeg. When cooked, let there be just a little surplus liquid; this will be absorbed by the one cup of precooked brown rice, which you finally add and heat all together.

Experimenting

Experiment according to your own taste. If you can leave potatoes — and perhaps bread too — out of your diet for just one month, eating brown rice instead whenever possible, you'll probably be surprised what it can do for you. If you find the rice constipating (but brown rice is less likely to give trouble in this respect than is white rice) then always use half rice and half lentils.

Meat Variations

If you want to use meat in this type of recipe, it must be said that beef doesn't go particularly well with lentils. Pork does, but pork is never recommended for a health or fitness diet. For one thing, porkmeat is too dense, heavy and fattening; and for another, it is not considered wholesome because pigs are not herbivorous but omnivorous — in plain English, they'll eat anything. The right meat for this particular purpose is lamb: shoulder, or stewing pieces, in approximately two-inch cubes should be cooked with a chopped onion, a little salt and a seasoning — preferably a few fresh leaves — of sweet basil. The meat will in any case take longer to cook than the lentils, so if you want to cook it first, chill it and remove the fat, that's okay. If you feel you do not need to do this, stew it for an hour or rather more, simply skim off the floating oil, and make sure there's enough liquid; then add the lentils, lemon juice and nutmeg. The pre-cooked rice of course is added last, or you could add a lesser quantity of raw brown rice to cook with the meat from the beginning.

If you make this with red lentils and leave out the rice,

you probably have a good approximation to the dish for which Esau sold his birthright (Genesis 25:29), according to the opinion of a number of biblical scholars and others who have tasted lamb and lentil stew.

Dietary Traps to Avoid

The following general list is of foods which should be avoided as far as possible by *everyone*. It is not meant as a complete list for the person who wants a strict weight-loss diet; it is intended even for the body builder, since the building of firm muscle must be accompanied by the paring away, or better still the avoidance, of fatty tissues. Unless you are on a strict diet, however, an occasional indulgence in one or more of these things will probably do no harm.

Alcoholic drinks, including "light" beers and wines.

Avocado, however prepared.

Carbonated drinks—never mind the calorie count, carbon dioxide has no calories but impairs the blood's functioning.

Cheeses, blue or processed

Cream, sweet or sour

Ice cream and all its elaborations

Mayonnaise and all "salad dressings". *Use* olive oil with cider vinegar

Pickles. Unsweetened dill pickle in moderation is okay if not over-brined

Pork and anything made from it

Pretzels, saltines, tortillas

Potato chips and fries

Processed meats of all kinds

Salted nuts, salted peanut butter, salted & buttered popcorn

Sausages, unless home made

Sauces and gravies, home made included*
Soft drinks, except pure fruit juices
Tobacco. Besides its well-known dangers to heart and
lungs, and its less well-known detriment to eyesight,
the use of tobacco perceptibly diminishes the sensitivity of a person's organs of taste and smell, this
resulting in over-seasoning of foods.

The above list is additional to other pointers given in
the text of this chapter. If, however, you exclude from your
usual diet all the things in this list only, your fitness and
your conscious awareness of fitness must be greatly enhanced thereby. Once the system is not encumbered with non-
nutrients including salt and sugar excesses, once damaging
substances are not being ingested (such as carbonated
drinks which put carbon dioxide into the blood in the same
way that the water we drink adds to the blood's supply of
oxygen) your fitness can rise to its natural and radiant
level.

Caffeine

Some people may be surprised that caffeine is not
included in the above list. If your doctor tells you to stop
drinking coffee, of course, you should stop.† For most

---

*The domestic custom of making a gravy for a roast by boiling up flour and water
with the fat from the meat, is not recommended. Several cooked unsweetened
fruits are traditional for use as sauces with meat, and a little experimentation
might lengthen the list. Besides the traditional applesauce with pork, pineapple
is finding wide acceptance in the western world. The red currant jelly which is
traditional with roast lamb in British custom, is simply the juice of red currants
squeezed from the fruit through a muslin bag, then left to set at room temperature by means of its own pectin. Plain stewed gooseberries, now served to
accompany roast duck, were probably served in earlier centuries with goose.
Cranberries were given their name by the Dutch, who regarded the crane as a
table bird. American language and custom retained the name, but transferred the
cranberry sauce to the turkey. The orange sauces which are served with roast
duck or with fried chicken are rather more complex, but need not be over-
elaborate. Following the same principle, the slice of lemon which is often served
with fish is to be preferred to *sauce tartare*.
†Some decaffeinated coffee has been demonstrated to contain dangerous substances as a result of its processing. Imitation coffees generally, made from burnt
barley and similar substances, do nothing for you but to impair the hot water you
mix them with, and most of them taste depressingly foul as well. A wide range of
interesting teas is now available, all of which contain less caffeine than coffee
does; some just naturally contain none. If you want to cut down on coffee, why
not experiment?

people there is probably no need for more than reasonable caution, not to overdo the intake of caffeine: hardly anyone can claim to be living at a completely natural tempo, and a little aid is probably not out of place for anyone in normal health.

However, it's as well to consider why you drink coffee, and when. If you just want to be sociable and join your friends in a cup of something, or if you want something to do as a reason to sit back from your work for a few minutes, or if you simply are thirsty, you'd be as well to join the large number of people these days who, for any of those reasons, would take a cup of hot water. (That will often give a person a slight and pleasant "lift", too.) If you need a cup of coffee as a booster towards the end of the day, or for a business meeting or so forth, then there's no reason why you should not use it for that purpose. But if you feel you need to keep drinking coffee *all day* to keep yourself alert or awake, then you are misinterpreting the signals and what you really need is something else.

There are a number of different possible causes of the trouble. Let's begin with the obvious one which is hardly ever mentioned: you may, just simply and genuinely, need more sleep.

Whether you have a problem or not, you might just take a look at your appointment book and ask yourself, if you suddenly decided you'd like a real early night, when is the soonest you could take it? If the answer is more than a week away, your schedule could use some pruning. Don't wait for over-fatigue to hit you!

If you don't lack time for sleep, stress could be your problem and coffee won't help that. Relaxation is likely to be what you need in that case.

Or it may be that you feel you could sleep the clock round and still feel tired. That could indicate a nutritional lack. In such a case coffee temporarily helps you draw further on your already depleted reserves, while what you need is the right thing to build them up. Check your diet to ensure you are getting the following foods frequently: Leafy green vegetables: raw, steamed or rapidly boiled. Bran (that's a good ingredient for your cereal mix). Milk (if you generally use skim milk, give so-called "whole milk" a whirl for a few weeks, or until you get this tiredness problem sorted out). Bananas (you might be surprised how important they can be in this problem). Mushrooms. Carrots. Peas, beans, lentils, brown rice, whole grain cereals, whole grain bread. Eggs. Real butter. If you eat meat, put the emphasis on liver, kidney and any other "organ meats" available, also clams and other fish: if you don't eat meat, then go all out for the milk, mushrooms, peas, beans, lentils and leafy greens. And cheddar cheese.

Some part of that diet probably will dispel the cause of the trouble. If it doesn't you might check with your doctor. The cause might be eyestrain or weak arches or anything in between, or it might just possibly be the sort of nutritional deficiency you ought not to handle yourself. Or your doctor might find nothing wrong with you. You may be needing to get energy from other sources.

Energy from Exercise

You need oxygen for energy, as you know: oxygen from the air you breathe into your lungs, from the air your skin breathes, and from the water you drink. The last one is looked after by making sure you drink plenty of good, unboiled water. If you want to drink hot water, you certainly don't need it boiling; if you want to make tea or coffee from water boiled in a kettle, remove it from the heat the moment it boils. A coffee-making machine uses the water immediately on boiling in any case.

The first two ways of getting oxygen are made more active by exercise, and exercise in the open air is obviously the most effective. If you work for a firm that has a fitness program — and fitness programs are on the increase now — go into that program enthusiastically. Never mind if you don't feel you can cope with it; that's the worry of the experts who are organizing these things. Your muscles need to limber up and to throw off any waste deposits which may have settled in them, and that new oxygen supply needs to circulate and take effect in your body. Those two factors work together. All you have to do — in fact, all you can do — is to put all the energy you have and all the goodwill you can into that program.

Even if you find your work itself boring — which may be one of the causes of your problem — a fitness program of that kind can make all the difference to that too, giving you a new interest, a new slant on the people you work with, a new kind of motivation.

Supposing there isn't such a program, see what you can do for yourself. Revise your personal exercise plan, and above all get into the open air whenever possible. In any case, keep up your Rhythmic Breathing and your good new plans for radiant fitness. They'll all work for you. And have green growing plants — "oxygen friends" — around you in your home.

Energy from Relaxation

In Chapter 5 the importance of the diaphragm in breathing was emphasized. Stress, tension, anxiety, oppose this action of the diaphragm. It becomes cramped and impedes the breathing; there is a tendency to hold the breath. Neck and scalp contract in sympathy with the diaphragm. The blood vessels in arms and legs contract. So one might literally "get cold feet", or might develop a tension headache. Anger can produce similar reactions: of one woman it was said that if ever she was seen warming her hands, it meant trouble for somebody!

Clearly it's of no use telling yourself (or another person in that state of tension) to "get a grip on yourself." You have a deadlock on yourself already.

Prolonged states of mild anxiety, extended and apparently accepted frustration, produce these same reactions, sometimes with such a gentle onset that the victim is quite unaware of the increasing muscular stiffness until maybe it becomes actually painful. And all that time he or she is suffering the effects of poor breathing, poor circulation, deficient sleep.

There is only one way to deal effectively with such a state of things if you realize you have developed it. The Deep Mind, remember, cannot be reasoned with nor, generally, approached directly. It has to be given an image of what's wanted, some kind of "presentation" of the desired effect.

In this case you present your image in the form of *acting, mime*. Words are not likely to be helpful, but if you can have a soft light and either some restful music or one of those nature-sound effects like rushing water, so much the better. The aim is to build an image of repose.

You lie down on the rug or some other flat, pleasant surface with nothing to raise your head. (If you can lie on a slantboard with your head slightly down, that's a help too; but the board would need to be long enough to extend your whole body, not just to the knees.) Lie in the "Earth Posture" described in Chapter 6 — palms up, sideways or down, just as you please — and establish your Rhythmic Breathing.

(If you are helping another person to relax in this way, someone who doesn't know about Rhythmic Breathing, just tell him or her to breathe as if pretending to be in a deep sleep. We've mostly taught ourselves how to do that, as children.)

Just lie quietly for a few moments; there's no rush.

Next, keeping up the Rhythmic Breathing, begin progressively to relax your body. Don't go straight to the center of the trouble, the solar plexus; start with your toes. If you simply "tell" them to relax, this may not work. The only contact your conscious mind has with your toes (or any other part of your body) is through the nervous system and its controlling power, your Deep Mind; and your Deep Mind has unaccustomed itself to obeying orders to relax. So give it a command it *will* accept, first. Tell those toes to clench tight. Then relax them, wriggle them around. Then relax them altogether.

Proceed to do the same thing with your ankles; then so up your whole body, step by step, first tightening then relaxing, using, relaxing each set of muscles in turn. Relaxing the abdominals is, for the present purpose, the critical point of the whole procedure. When you come to your arms, relax each one separately, beginning with the fingers; then follow the method very thoroughly for your neck and face. When you come to relax your face, make it very calm, with the sense of a slight smile. Your Deep Mind will register the feeling appropriate to that action, because it has such a close habitual link with facial expression.

Don't forget your neck and scalp. You can effectively move your neck muscles by raising your head a few inches from the ground, then slowly lowering it. If you have learned to twitch your ears or to move your scalp back and forth, you'll have no problem with your scalp; otherwise, simply *try* to move it. (If, after this session of relaxation is over, your scalp is tight, move it back and forth with your fingertips, changing the positions of your two hands after each group of about five movements, up to a total of at least thirty or forty movements. If you can have a friend do this for you, you'll be able to relax even better.)

After relaxing every part of your body, check over, mentally, from your toes up, to make sure it has stayed relaxed. For any part which has clenched up in tension again, go through the same procedure as before: clench even tighter, then relax, use and move the muscles, and then relax again. When relaxation is really complete, lie still and enjoy it for at least fifteen minutes.

How Relaxation Increases Energy

Relaxation gives you increased energy in several ways. To begin with, it "gives" you the energy which would otherwise be used up in needlessly and painfully tensing all your muscles. Besides this, by restoring normal mobility to your diaphragm and your intercostal muscles (the muscles between your ribs), it "unlocks" your breathing and allows you to take a good supply of air into your lungs. Then relaxation allows your blood vessels to return to normal, instead of being compressed and contracted — those cold hands and feet! — so that your blood again circulates as it should, removing waste products from every muscle and organ and revitalizing them with fresh, oxygenated blood. Your nerves themselves are cleansed and nourished in the process, so that they convey messages more readily to and from your brain, and from one part to another of the sympathetic system. This means that your brain, your heart, and even your digestive organs are able to do their work more rapidly and more effectively; you are better nourished, better rested and renewed, better supplied with oxygen, and all for less effort.

Energy and Meditation

The practice of meditation has long been recognized as conferring great psychic and even bodily benefits. Much research has been done in recent years upon the "how" and "why" of this, and since the work has been pursued by many methods and has been prompted by a diversity of initial questions, the massive resulting evidence in many respects lacks correlation. However, here is a summary of a few points derived from it which should be of value to you in pursuit of psycho-physical fitness.

What Meditation Is and Is Not

True meditation develops into an altered state of consciousness. It is *not* "meditating about" this or that, which generally means a chain of intellectual cogitations; although any material object or non-material idea can focus the mind as a starting point for meditation. These days, true meditation is frequently called "transcendental meditation" because it is said to transcend the intellectual state. On the evidence, however it mught just as well be said to undercut the rational process, or, better still, simply to be other than it: simply to be true meditation. It is in fact a very natural, perhaps primal state of awareness.

This may make meditation more acceptable to many people. To meditate genuinely, effectively and beneficially, it is certainly not required that you should try to force yourself into the world of pure mind or into the world of Deity: still less into the limitless realms of selfless abstraction. All of these concepts have haunted the idea of meditation for innumerable people, whether they look at the Eastern or at the Western schools. If you are at a high level of spiritual evolution, your meditation will be elevated thereby. If you are not, perseverence in the practice of meditation will certainly elevate you, but without pain or reluctance on your part. Research has shown that even statistics of crime drop where true meditation is practiced, nor is this surprising; meditation breaks the hold upon the psyche of those abnormal cultural stresses which frequently drive people to act contrary to their better judgement.

Mystics and the Natural World

Great spiritual leaders and mystics — who in the

nature of things are of all people least ashamed of their common humanity — have consistently been great meditators. They have also consistently manifested a great sense of being "at home" with the world of nature. The Buddha's universal compassion, and the Prophet Muhammad's happy relationship with the animals that came into his life — not to forget his acknowledgment of the ants as "a people" — are two interestingly contrasted examples of this feeling. The saintly woman mystic, Rabi'a, exemplified that aspect in the Moslem spirit most strongly. The discourses of the Christ contain a remarkable number of references to the plant world: the lilies of the field, the fields ripe for harvest, the grain of mustard seed, the parable of the sower, and more; while the man held by millions of people to have been the greatest exponent of Christianity since apostolic times — St. Francis of Assisi — is renowned above all for his wholehearted sincerity in naming all living beings, and the splendors of the heavens, as his brothers and sisters.

Non-intellectual Awareness and Your Blood Pressure

For all of us, this affinity between meditative awareness and communion with the world of nature, has important connotations in the area of psycho-physical fitness. *By whichever means you approach the "primal" type of non-intellectual, non-verbal consciousness — which may be an "older-brain" consciousness — researches have shown it to be conducive to the lower levels of stress, lower levels of blood pressure.*

Research indicates that whenever we speak to another human being — a family member or whoever — there is some increase, however slight, in our blood pressure. It seems any verbal encounter with other humans is recognized as a potential threat or challenge, demanding either verbal thinking or the expression (or disguise) of a non-verbal emotion or concept by means of words. Even an adult speaking to a child can have stressful doubts as to how much to say, or how the words will be interepreted.

When we speak to animals — again, on the research findings — this rise in blood pressure does not occur; in fact, emotional stress and physical tension are reduced. That is part of the reason why the company of even one animal is now being widely recognized as bringing such high therapeutic good (and so much undemanding love) into the lives of lonely children, invalids, the elderly, anyone living through a traumatic experience or with the scar of one. Even having plants to tend helps people in similar ways. Although we may indeed speak in words to either animal or plant, we know inwardly that the words as such mean nothing to them: it is the emotional-instinctual tone underlying the words, which they respond to. These day-by-day contacts with the world of nature can be, for all of us, time spent in an "Eden" of innocence, an unchanged Golden Age, where the subrational and the suprarational in us can meet and merge without need of differentiation. There, with neither explanation nor apology required, we can walk relaxed and carefree in that most difficult of all nudities to attain, nudity of soul.

Meditation can bring us a similar kind of release from our own and other people's cogitations: the findings are that it can bring us similar, even intensified, positive benefits to both psyche and body. (Further comparison might well be unfair, however, for meditation has certainly been subjected to thorough investigations which most likely have never been accorded to life in communion with the world of nature.)

Some Demonstrated Benefits of Meditation

Research indicates that meditation improves people's circulation (by relaxing stress-related contraction of the blood vessels and even weakened heart action from the same cause), increasing the supply of blood to the brain. This enhances the mental powers, and facial youthfulness.

By focusing attention in another manner and upon another object, meditation automatically suspends worry, thereby weakening its hold over the consciousness: and release from worry is another great rejuvenator of both the psyche and the body.

And, as has been indicated, meditation tends to lower blood pressure which has been above normal, and thus to lengthen life.

Furthermore, meditation aids strong and right development of moral character — that is, of truly free choice — by giving the psyche escape, if only for brief periods, from those social pressures and artificial values which, so long as they seem permanent and omnipotent, have power to drive people either into servile evasion or into defiance.

It remains to indicate some of the ways in which a condition of true meditation, and its consequent altered state of consciousness, may be achieved.

Ways into meditation: The Mantram

Assume the Egyptian posture (see Chapter 5 for description) or any other alert but comfortable posture in which you can sit still and forget your body. Establish your Rhythmic Breathing, and remain thus until you feel completely settled and ready to begin.

Take a word, preferably one which is very familiar to you: "sky", "hurry", "apple", "yellow", or anything you please. Some people can use this method well by using their own name. On each out-breath, say this word aloud, slowly and distinctly in an even, unvarying tone.

Your first meditation session might be for twenty minutes, but you can gradually lengthen subsequent sessions up to forty-five; that means that the whole session will be included within an hour. That is quite sufficient time for an unmonitored meditation, and in fact as you gain more practice you will be surprised how intense, yet profoundly refreshing, an experience it is. Meditate at least on alternate days, daily if possible. Your first session, and

perhaps several sunsequent ones, will doubtless be filled
with ideas which suggest themselves to you at every repetition of the chosen word. That is not "meditation", but is a
necessary preliminary stage. (When one you've chosen a
word, don't consider changing it for at least three months.)

Whatever trains of associated ideas the word raises in
your mind, don't follow any of them out; just keep on
repeating the same word in the same way. For success in
this method, a time should come when the sound of the
word becomes entirely dissociated from its meaning. If it is
your name that you have chosen as a mantram, it should
now seem inconceivable to you — while you are meditating — that that succession of sounds should mean "you".
But don't think, while meditating, even about this! You now
have your Mantram.

During your subsequent meditations, continue to pro
nounce that word aloud on every out-breath, slowly and
distinctly in an even, unvarying tone. (You'll find the tone
varies slightly from meditation to meditation. That is natural and need not disturb you.) Keep your mind on the
sound of the word: probably it will evoke no further images
or associations in your mind, but if it should do so, ignore
them. *Entertain no thought, no disturbing emotion. Thus you will
develop a state of true meditation, a state more peaceful even than
the varying levels of sleep. Gradually, with practice, you will
become aware of your "self feeling" — an indescribably peaceful
happiness which is not an "emotion", since an "emotion" is something which moves a person, and this, as you center in upon it,
stills you.*

*To mark the close of your meditation session, the ideal is to
have a reliable friend to call you gently at a pre-arranged time. Failing this, you should have an electric, quartz or anyway silent alarm
clock somewhere to hand where it will not be visible to you, and set
it for the close of your meditation. The essential thing is, to have
some completely trustworthy arrangement so that you, meditating,*

*can put the thought of time right out of your mind, and can dismiss
it if it occurs to you.* *

Ways into Meditation: Music

For many people, who have been impressed from an
early age with the idea that words and thought were insep-
arably linked, meditation by the mantram method may
prove virtually impossible to achieve. If you have this difficulty, or if you wish to experience a number of methods,
try using suitable sound.

If you use music, you need a reflective and repetitive
piece. If you or a friend understand the matter, you could
have a "loop" tape made of the most meditative portion of
your chosen piece, so you can listen to it without interruption throughout your meditation time. Music you might
consider for this purpose includes such pieces as Pachel-
bel's "Canon", the "Pavane for a Dead Princess" by Ravel.
Or Handel's "Largo" might appeal to you if it has no particularly strong associations for you.

A good and interesting alternative to music for this
purpose is some form of natural sound. You might use a
tape of birdsong in the same way as the music tape, or any
form of "white noise" — sounds of surf, a stream, a waterfall
— either on a tape or on a specialized synthesizer such as a
"Sound Conditioner", if you have one.

Use any gentle sound which appeals to you. Only, as
with the mantram, when you have made your choice keep
to the one thing for at least three months. (If you wish to use

---

* It may be noted, with regard to the Mantram method, that teachers who adhere to
some particular religious or metaphysical system commonly instruct their pupils to
use as a mantram some word or succession of sounds which has a particular
significance in that system; thus we find the use of Aum, Jai, Shalom, and of a
number of sacred names. The teachers may wish to inspire the pupils through
the necessary perseverance of the early stages in this way, or perhaps to link the
bliss of the ultimate self-feeling with their own system. Certainly there is no
reason why you should not, if you wish, use as your mantram a word which has
high spiritual associations for you, but such is not needed for the success of this
method of meditation, which depends, as does every method, ultimately upon
clearing the mind and not upon filling it.

a mantram for three months or longer, a sound for three months or longer, and the other ways into meditation which will be mentioned, each for three months or longer, it will *probably* delay your progress to the deeper levels of meditation somewhat, but you will gain some worthwhile experiences and an inner understanding of the differences.)

Conduct and conclude your meditation as indicated in the italicised portions of the preceding section on *The Mantram*. As with the word, you may find your first few sessions are filled with associated ideas, but the verbal formulations should clear more quickly.

Don't let yourself "think in words" while you listen to music or sound. If you are one before whose "inner eye" scenes pass while you listen to music, avoid attaching either words or rationalizations to the scenes. "See" them and let them go. If you are one who "sees" formless clouds of color while listening, that's fine. Enjoy them — but avoid thinking about them, or naming or identifying them. Let your peripheral consciousness immerse itself in their bright splendor, but keep your attention centrally upon the sound. When the associations have all passed away, you have your meditation experience.

Ways Into Meditation: The Yantra

Gazing at an abstract geometrical pattern is for some folk the key to meditation. In India, custom has established the use of a pattern having a profound metaphysical interpretation, such a pattern being termed a *Yantra*. So long as the figure is regular, balanced and harmonious, and is fairly intricate, there is no need for it to have any special significance. You should not in fact look for one, nor should you turn your pattern into a mathematical puzzle. A good thing to use, if you can get hold of it, is one of those boldly printed black and white designs — whether spiral or other — which usually are placed upon a revolving device for purposes of hypnotism. You will not be revolving it.

Your design should in any case be boldly executed, and should be large enough to be used for its intended purpose in complete relaxation.

With your design secured vertically to a wall facing you, or held on your thighs and slightly sloped for easy vision, begin and conclude your meditation in accordance with the italicized portions in the section on *The Mantram*. Let your eyes follow the lines as they will, only avoid *thinking about* the pattern or about anything else. Keep bringing back your attention to the pattern itself as often as may be necessary, patiently but persistently. The time will come when your mind will know, when you sit down and gaze at that pattern, you mean meditation. Then it will stop trying to entertain you with ideas about the pattern, and you have your meditation symbol.

So Meditate!

Meditation — switching off your thinking machinery — for forty-five minutes every day or on alternate days — is more than worth the initial efforts you may put into it. In fact, the greater effort you find it to sit still and stop thinking during your meditation time, the more seriously you need it.

It is more relaxing and refreshing even than a great deal of our sleep is, since for many people the stresses and intellection processes of the waking life don't entirely cut out during sleep as they should.

Think of it if you like as a brief but intensive trip into the wilds — into the unspoiled territory of your own inner nature. It's always there waiting for you, no matter how ravaged and hassled you may feel by outer-world happenings or by your own emotions.

You will find, too, that besides all the direct benefits from meditation which were indicated earlier, that when after meditation you return to the use of words and to the processes of your rational mind, you will be able to think more clearly and more logically; because (1) you will perceive more easily what is the point towards which you are directing your thinking — a point which in many instances never does get expressed in words because it remains in the wordless domain of the will — and (2) because you will learn to distinguish more clearly between your thoughts and your feelings, both of which are necessary components of your psychic life, but neither of which should be either allowed or expected to do the work of the other.

So meditate! Your radiant fitness will flourish and shine forth, your outer life will be enriched, as the psychically and physically cramping burden of stress is lifted from you. *Never was a more glorious reward offered for sitting and doing nothing.*

Summing Up on Nourishment and Energy
(1) Energy Gained by Material Means

Energy comes to us from the food we eat, from the air we breathe (through lungs and skin), from the water we drink. Eating good food is not enough: for radiant fitness we have to avoid clogging the tissues of our bodies with toxic or inert non-foods, to avoid clogging our blood stream with substances which impede its life giving work for our vital organs.

Exercise steps up our energy by increasing our oxygen intake and by improving the circulation of the blood. (It may also give a healthier appetite, and certainly can save a lot of wasted effort and the carrying of dead weight, by limbering and firming the muscles and helping in the dispersion of fat.)

Relaxation positively gives us more energy by allowing the diaphragm and chest muscles to function better, improving the breathing, and it improves the circulation and heart action by removing constriction from the blood vessels and the muscles. (Remember — the heart is a muscle.)

In some cases, stress impairs digestion or the functioning of the whole alimentary system; relaxation is a necessary factor in adjusting that too.

(2) Energy Gained by Non-Material Means

Meditation enhances the value of ordinary relaxation, and does more besides. Developed meditation gives us experience of our true selves, essentially free, essentially peaceful, *essentially happy.* When we know *by experience* that we have an inner reality to which all the troubles and stresses of life are external, we may be earnest, concerned, committed, but we never need let things "get us down" again. Earnestness, concern, commitment are *voluntary* (they couldn't be virtues otherwise); being "got down", driven, stressed by anxiety are involuntary, negative conditions and are of no use to anyone. Meditation helps us keep our overview, our sense of proportion, and that inner radiance which will shine forth and cause people to bless our presence in times of trouble.

As earlier chapters have shown, we can gain energy also from sources which, although they are perceptible to us as parts of the material universe, yet do not communicate their energy to us as food, or as fuel, or by electric wires. We gather such energy from the planetary and zodiacal powers, from the earth currents, from trees. Psychically — and physically too in a subtle way — we are part of an invisible network of energy sources from which, if we do not shut outselves off, we shall draw whatever we need. Openness, receptivity is all.

Will others not draw from us according to their needs? Certainly! — but we never need be left depleted. If we feel we are not replenished by the natural leveling tendency of the system, there is always your overhead Center (Chapter 3), representing the Light of your Higher Self upon which you can draw at any time. There are no barriers to our replenishment unless we create them.

The secret of life is the exchange of energies. The secret of love is the exchange of energies. The secret of Tao is the exchange of energies. Stagnation is death. Miserliness, at whatever level, is death. Circulation is life: it is life at the physical level, at the astral, mental, and at the highest spiritual level of being. For life, for health, for spiritual vitality and for radiant fitness, keep the channels open for circulation and exchange of energies.

Author's Note

In case you desire information or supplies in the areas of nutrition and exercise, and do not know where to find what you want, the following firms are mentioned for their specialized practical knowledge, fair dealing and reasonable prices. Both supply to mail order:

General Nutrition Corporation, 418 Wood Street, Pittsburgh, PA 15222-1878

Vitamin and mineral dietary supplements, some specifically from non-meat sources; weight gain and loss formulae, pollen, amino acids etc; with a number of health foods, health and fitness aids, skin and scalp care products. Their catalog gives helpful facts and notes on current research trends.

Health for Life, 8033 Sunset Blvd. Suite 483, Los Angeles, CA 90046

Exercise regimens for healthy muscle building, body sculpture and suppleness, for men and women, using minimal/optional equipment; also a sane, and guaranteed, weight loss plan. These people impress with their recognition of the need for harmony of action, not only within the body but also between body and mind.

Chapter Nine

MEANWHILE THE MIND

Meanwhile, the mind from pleasure less
Withdraws into its happiness:
The mind, that ocean where each kind
Does straight its own resemblance find;
Yet it creates, transcending these,
Far other worlds and other seas . . .

> *Andrew Marvell, "Thoughts in a Garden"*

And am I wrong to worship where
Faith cannot doubt, nor hope despair,
Since my own soul can grant my prayer?
Speak, God of Visions, plead for me
And tell why I have chosen thee!

> *Emily Bronte, "Plead for Me"*

The mirror, whether of glass, steel, silver or bronze, has been recognized through the ages as an instrument whose potential goes far beyond satisfying the brief concern of vanity.

In some ways the mirror resembles its relative, the crystal sphere, as a "window" between dimensions of being. The sphere, to be sure, is the better known instrument for the psychic perception of other times and regions, and has also been employed to hold a visualized image with which psychic work is to be done. Mirrors too, however, have been employed for all these purposes. Not only clairvoyance and past life recall, but powerful love spells, defense spells for deflecting a "cross" or a "hex", explorations of the unseen worlds, and much good healing work, have been, and are, performed with the aid of gazing-crystals and mirrors alike.

But This is Easy!

The kind of psychic work with mirrors which will be described here, and which you can perform — to the great help and furtherance of your program for radiant fitness — is simpler and easier than these, and does not call for the expertise or the long concentrated practice required by some of them. Even the visualizations are so simple and natural, you need hardly realize you are doing them. (Which is not surprising, since you probably visualize all the time and hardly, if at all, realize you are doing it!)

Your Mirror(s)

One is necessary, two are better. You may use several. For this type of psychic work there's no need that a mirror should be specially prepared or dedicated in any way. It is very desirable, however, that at least one of the mirrors should be used exclusively by you and not shared with any other person. We shall call this your personal mirror.

A "traveling mirror" — rectangular, about four inches by six, and of either glass or metal — can if need be serve very well as the personal mirror, particularly as you can carry it with you. The customary little round, purse-size mirror which shows about one and one-half features at a time is practically useless for this kind of mirror work, although it can be quite effective for other kinds. Even here, the more experienced practitioner might find it useful to give herself an encouraging grin, or a morale-boosting wink, in the course of a stressful day. But the larger rectangular mirror is of more substantial worth, and besides, could find a place in the gear of male seekers for radiant fitness too.

The next size of mirror to be considered is the head-and-shoulders mirror. This is likely to be a dresser mirror, and, as such, will appeal to many people as a personal mirror, partly because a dresser is frequently the territory of one specific person, and partly because this is the mirror at which you can sit down and get on friendly terms with your reflection.

It will not appeal to everyone, however; either because their household arrangements are different, or because the depth of the dresser — the double depth of the dresser, since you have to look across both it and its reflection before you come to *your* reflection — creates such a barrier of distance. In either of these cases, a wall mirror either in bedroom or dressing room may be the personal mirror.

(If you want to keep a personal mirror quite private, get a picture-framer to put a piece of plastic mirror in the back of the frame of a picture.)

The third size of mirror for you to consider is almost a necessity, even though, unless you live alone, it's most unlikely you'll be able to claim this as your personal mirror. This is the full length mirror. From the viewpoint of your fitness program, it's far better to look at yourself full length from time to time in a mirror shared with the rest of the family (it's far better to look at yourself full length, even, in a gymnasium mirror at the same time as twenty other people) than never to look at yourself full length at all.

If you have a traveling mirror which can move around with you, a head-and-shoulders mirror, and (on whatever terms) a full length mirror, you are well equipped for the psychic mirror work of radiant fitness. One of the three will be your special, personal mirror, your "magical" mirror; but all of them will do good work for you.

Of Mirrors and Men

Tradition and literature have not, until this century, given fair treatment to men using mirrors. The myth of Narcissus probably began from the primitive fear that one's soul could be "snared" in a reflecting surface, the idea that Narcissus "fell in love" with his reflection being a later Greek fantasy; but there the story stands, one glance in the "mirror" was fatal. Euripides has only a passage — in "Hippolytus" — about Time holding up a mirror to the face of the evil man, whereupon he marvels at his own ugliness: a figure of speech which may have given Wilde the idea for *The Portrait of Dorian Gray*. The man referred to by the apostle James fares a little better, but not much: for having looked at himself in a mirror, he walks away and at once forgets what he looks like. (James 1:23-24). Certainly in Eastern and Gaelic lore alike, there have been male gazers in prophetic mirrors, but they seem to have gained little good by it. The story of Macbeth being shown the vision of the subsequent kings of Scotland, although a spurious "legend", is a typical sample.

Lastly, in Bram Stoker's "Dracula" — first published in 1897 — when Jonathan Harker has observed in his shaving mirror that the Vampire Count casts no reflection, Dracula simply hurls the offending glass out of the window, exclaiming "It is a foul bauble of man's vanity! Away with it!"

Only when we reach the first part of the present century, with "Strongfortism", Charles Atlas and the beginnings of the modern body-sculpture movement, do we find an awareness that for men as well as for women, the mirror has much to offer as a means of attaining what is desired in the way of physique and fitness. Then, among the "secrets" of the super-physique courses, men begin to be told *"Do your exercises in front of a mirror: watch your muscles in action."* But we shall return to that point.

Your Own Reflection: How Much Can It Do For You?

The limits of what your mirror image can do for you, depend altogether on the strength of the relationship you establish with it!

To understand the force of this statement, it is necessary to consider first another psychic technique which requires a considerably greater amount of preparation and practice.

That technique is called "The Formula of the Simulacrum". In this, a person who is practiced in giving forth astral substance, exteriorizes enough of it to form a life-size "image" of the physical presence, standing facing him or her and about ten feet away.

This "image", the Simulacrum, is then addressed in a positive, firm but totally loving manner, as one might address a younger sister or brother, on whatever topic the operator may consider her or his Deep Mind needs guidance. The Simulacrum is treated entirely as a representative of the Deep Mind. A person having a difficulty about stopping smoking, for example, may have tracked down the cause of his or her particular problem, and may tell the Simulacrum that certainly it's great to feel mature and adult, but to have clean lungs and to follow one's true will is far more mature and adult than smoking is. Never mind the pictures on the ads, which can only flatter the immature.

Or a person who overeats through anxiety might offer a bargain to the Simulacrum: "The thing I'm anxious about has nothing whatever to do with food shortage (or with eating up to please an angry Mom, or whatever may have been traced as the root of the Deep Mind's confused reactions). But, since you don't have the responsibility of coping with my problems, it's only fair I stop sending these worries down the wires to you. Henceforth I'll practice relaxation regularly, and keep from harrassing you with matters which are not part of your job, and you on your side will respond by letting up on the eating." Whatever is amiss is sorted out with the Simulacrum, and the desired instructions are given to it with assurances of love and confidence. The Simulacrum is next dispersed again into a formless cloud of astral substance. It is then re-absorbed *along with its programming,* so this becomes part of the programming of the Deep Mind. The dream life as well as the waking life are thereafter watched for the Deep Mind's reactions.

Those are just typical uses which people make of the Formula of the Simulacrum. It is a highly effective and potent technique, avoiding the coercions of hypnosis, gaining its object through building the natural relationship between the levels of the psyche to greater degrees of understanding and confidence. Clearly, this is the type of technique you can use to promote your general well-being and to enhance your radiant fitness; the only difficulty being to achieve the power to create the Simulacrum.

But you have your Simulacrum, there, looking at you from your mirror! — your own perfect image in reflected light. You can use that in a similar way, treating it as the representative of your Deep Mind and thus conveying to your Deep Mind your desires, aspirations, anything you want its immense powers to achieve for you. (But never forget, your Deep Mind for all its wondrous powers is younger brother or sister to your rational consciousness, while your Higher Self is, by far, the "Senior Partner" over both of you!)

The only difference in technique is that as you can't *re-absorb* your mirror image, you need to employ another method to make sure your Deep Mind really accepts, as addressed to it, the messages you give to your mirror image. That, in fact, presents no problem. You can organize things so your Deep Mind will be happy to make that identification.

Meeting Your Mirror Friend

In the first phase of this practice, don't concern yourself with your image anywhere but in your chosen personal mirror. Mirror images of you elsewhere are just "reflections"; you are not making anything of them. Later, you'll be able to choose whether to make something special of one of those other images, or not. At present you'll concentrate on forming a link between your Deep Mind and the image of you in the particular place you have specified, your personal mirror.

To begin with, take care to think and feel that your mirror friend is *someone*, a nice person who really feels friendly towards you but who looks to you to do the thinking and talking. Identify your image in your personal mirror with your "lower self", the emotional-instinctual part of you which is "animated" by your Deep Mind.

Make it a special point, every morning as soon as you can after getting up, to look in your personal mirror and give your mirror friend a smile and a greeting. Just a brief "Hi!" or "Hullo!" will do. Soon you can extend this, as and when you feel it's appropriate, with a little comment on some shared experience: "That storm was quite something!" or "Didn't we have a great dream!"

Your Deep Mind really wants to be friends with you, really wants to be in closer communication with you. When, as a regular thing, you address a warm feeling, friendly looks, communication, to the image in your personal mirror, your Deep Mind is not going to miss out on that. Your Deep Mind will get into line for the handouts, and will willingly identify with that mirror image. Don't expect to see any startling difference, but that's when your mirror friend "comes alive".

Talking To Your Mirror Friend

That's only the beginning. Remember, you have another technique also for creating a link-up of communication between your rational consciousness and your Deep Mind; that is, through your Rhythmic Breathing.

So, when you want to talk to your mirror friend and really make sure the message gets through, sit or stand in front of your personal mirror, establish your Rhythmic Breathing, give your mirror friend a real warm smile, and begin. You don't have to stand on ceremony. This is your impulsive, wayward kid brother/sister. Only this kid has a fantastic computer and is into all kinds of mysterious things, and in all love and friendship you'd appreciate some helpful co-operation.

Your Deep Mind is in any case not much inclined to verbal conversation, so there's no point in your saying a great deal. If you have a *picture* (maybe something from a magazine) which shows what you want by way of agility, strength, grace, happiness — "Here's how I want to be, wouldn't that be great for you too?" — or a race or contest, camp, stadium or wherever — "Here's *where* I want to be, will you help us both get there?" that could be enough to implant the right feeling, while you resume your Rhythmic Breathing and dwell upon your daydream. Your mirror friend will not be persuaded to help you by means of logical arguments, the *feeling* is everything.

You may get the impression that nothing much happens in these sessions where you confide to your mirror friend your aspiration to be a rock-climber or a dancer, a long distance runner or the fit and youthful mother of a family. In fact, the resultant co-ordination of attitudes between the conscious and unconscious levels of your psyche is of great importance.

Unexpected Reactions

Even while you sit or stand there, formulating and

imagining your heart's desire, you may pick up some immediate emotional responses from your mirror friend: perhaps enthusiastic concurrence with your ideas, or possibly something negative which may even come as a surprise to you.

— Is that what I really want?

We do, certainly, need to revise our daydreams and aspirations sometimes, and it is easy to go on imagining we still want something until confronted with the possibility of getting it. One remembers Scarlett O'Hara, who spent her life pursuing one particular man, only to turn him down at the last. But while you are examining this doubt, you should just check that it isn't disguising one of these others.

— Supposing I try, and fail?

In few endeavors is "failure" absolute. Even if you don't quite make your own high standards in your chosen sport, avocation or career, just simply doing the thing you feel you are "meant" to do can immensely enhance your life, and other people will be far more encouraged thereby than by the soaring of a quite inaccessible star. In such matters, the only lamentable "failure" would be failure to make the effort.

There is one case, however, in which the odds should be carefully weighed: that is the situation in which a happy and successful amateur in some sport has the daydream of being a great professional. There you have to consider not only the price of failure but, even more acutely, the price of success. There is an element of stagecraft in all professionalism, and the public does not generally see the damaged bodies and wrecked health of many of its idols. Are the laurels worth that gamble? The young aspirant is at liberty to answer "Yes", but the question should always be considered.

— How much effort and responsibility am I undertaking?

Predictably, plenty. Whatever we do in life, we are

"forever climbing up the climbing wave". Predictably, too, if you are doing what you want to do, you'll love it. Only two things are ever tedious: one is having too little to do, the other is having nothing congenial in the schedule. So go all out for your dreams.

— But I don't deserve to succeed!

That is a thing which people don't often say, even to themselves, but they let it haunt them all the same. If you detect such a feeling lurking in the shadows among your thoughts and emotions, try to pull it out into the light and look at it. Chances are you don't feel guilty *about* any particularly terrible thing (which anyway is irrelevant); most of the vague sense of "unworthiness" which hinders some people from following their aspirations is simply a kind of self-disappointment. Perhaps one of the best ways to deal with this is to realize that what you are looking at is mostly a collection of raw materials — the tacky palette of paints, the kitchen table littered with ingredients, the workbench with tools, blueprints, pieces of metal and other materials in the midst of being shaped and assembled. Nobody likes such things to come under the gaze of a critical eye; so don't turn that critical gaze on the busy studio, kitchen, workshop of your own self in the making!

Forgive Yourself!

For anything beyond that — blunders, mistakes, things you may regret having done or having neglected — it's important to forgive yourself. It's of no use for people to talk about an "all-merciful God" and then refusing, as so many people do, to forgive themselves.

It has sometimes been said that all refusal to forgive oneself springs from a misplaced pride or vanity: refusal to forgive oneself for being less than perfect. Undoubtedly there is some truth in that, but it is not the whole truth. For one thing, a great deal of guilt feeling is traceable to *fear of retribution;* not only of retribution for whatever wrong one may initially have done, but also of retribution for not feeling guilty, if one doesn't.

Now, this is to mistake a human characteristic for a divine or karmic one. We see all the time, if a person has done something of which his or her associates disapprove — no matter if it has in no wise harmed them, and if it is none of their business — how assiduously they will try, sometimes in quite subtle ways, to ensure that that person will be made to feel guilty. They are frequently not aiming for that person's punishment, which would have a beginning and an end, but just to make his or her life unhappy.

Whether you conceive of the Divine authority in your life as God, Karma or your Higher Self, you should realize when you reflect deeply about it that he, she or it doesn't operate in that way! How could anyone ever evolve spiritually if they were to be continually brought back to their weakest moments? The call is always to progress, to advance, to dissociate oneself from past errors — when, indeed, they were errors. The important thing is that we should see quite honestly in our own mind where our offbeat actions came from — faulty judgment, silly blunder, or the only rational way to cope with maybe an irrational situation. The best course then is to go out and take a look at the night sky, or at some other grand and immense natural phenomenon, and be refreshed by the realization of the tiny scale of all our concerns. Forgive yourself? Yes, of course! Wipe the slate clean for yourself, straighten your shoulders and start over. W.B. Yeats caught the spirit of it, to conclude his "Dialogue of Self and Soul"—

> I am content to follow to its source
> Every event in action as in thought,
> Measure the lot, forgive myself the lot!
> When such as I cast out remorse,
> So great a sweetness flows into the breast

We must laugh and we must sing,
We are blest by everything,
Everything we look upon is blest.

When You are Your Own Victim

There is a completely different type of situation in which people sometimes find self-forgiveness difficult, and that is in the painful experience of having to suffer for one's own folly, forgetfulness or inaction. One might for instance carelessly lose or break a treasured possession, something not easily replaced, and one might feel one can never forgive oneself for that loss.

There are several ways to look at this. From an ideal spiritual viewpoint, it might be said no material object is worth that much; that the loser should remember Blake's lines —

He who kisses the joy as it flies
Lives in Eternity's sunrise.

But we don't always feel willing or able to kiss our joys as they fly. We may feel acutely that at our present stage of evolution, some particular thing is an intrinsic part of our life. That which is lost may indeed be a material object — some beautiful treasured possession which, from whatever cause, is gone — or it may be a bodily faculty lost as the result of sickness or accident.

If something of any of these kinds should befall you, you should certainly "let go", if you feel that's possible for you, and learn a valuable spiritual lesson therefrom. It *is* good to be able to live perpetually in anticipation of the adventure of tomorrow, never looking back. But you are by no means morally bound to take this attitude, and if you don't feel able to do so, it is better to be honest with yourself than to have a hidden, perhaps completely repressed regret. At the same time, you can — and should — forgive yourself for what has occurred.

There is a confusion here which many people have with regard to their attitude to others, and it can apply equally well to your attitude to yourself. It is mentioned here because if you don't understand it, it can at some time damage your relationship with your Deep Mind.

Forgiveness and Justice

If you forgive a person who, let's say, has robbed you, you are still entitled to get your property back. You can forgive, you can claim the return of your property, you can even consent to the punishment of the culprit for some good reason — not personal vindictiveness — and your forgiveness can still be perfectly genuine and sincere; as, in fact, it could not be if your sense of justice were outraged.

(So, too, if you have wronged some other person in a way in which restitution is possible, you should make that resitution to the best of your ability but you should also forgive yourself. Making restitution is in fact part of the "forgiving" process, making the incident as if it hadn't happened.)

All this has applications in your relationship with your Deep Mind. You should realize your Deep Mind is not particularly aware of justice as such; that is a concern of your rational consciousness, and of your Higher Self. If you've come to grief through some piece of absent-mindedness or laziness, or through yielding to a foolish impulse, it's of no more use to *blame* your Deep Mind than to blame a pet dog or a baby. But your Deep Mind — unlike the pet dog or the baby — can reasonably be called upon to do something about it.

So don't ever say, or think, "I'll never forgive myself for being so foolish! Your Deep Mind is the recipient of this unforgiveness, and, as the past cannot in that sense be undone, you are setting up an irremediable and therefore potentially neurotic situation.

Be patient, be positive, be constructive. Give your Deep Mind a way to repair the blunder.

Claiming the Help of Your Deep Mind

Whether you want, as suggested above, to put right something out of the past, or are looking entirely to a new development in the future, you can call upon your Deep Mind, with its very extensive powers, to help you.

For one thing, of course, you can and should establish your Rhythmic Breathing, and tell your resolve — it should not be less than a resolve — to your mirror friend, as representative of your Deep Mind. But, to make particularly sure of engaging your Deep Mind in this matter, you should employ another means as well, and one which will also have reference to your mirror friend.

It is essential — and particularly in the early stages of any practice intended to involve the Deep Mind — that your approach should be

specific

dramatic

systematic.

Specific, to allow of no possible doubt as to what you want; and no possible doubt that you want it.

Dramatic, to engage the imagination and to ensure the interest of the Deep Mind in furthering your project.

Systematic, to bring your project within the ambit of Time, out of the realms of fantasy, and to engage the Deep Mind in a schedule.

The Wishing Tree

Achieving a wish, a dream, an aspiration, is somewhat like climbing a tree.

No two trees are exactly alike.

Every tree presents its particular snags, obstacles, weak or isolated branches, spiky growths in which you could become entangled.

Every tree offers its particular footholds, handholds, easy slopes and forks to help you on your way.

Every tree offers its reward: the view from the summit, or a leafy palace in which to rest and meditate, or a paradise of blossom, or sweet fruit or nuts that you can eat, with some to throw down to your friends.

But there are times for doing those things. You want to climb during the good weather, you want the right season for the leaves, the blossoms, the fruit: you need a clear day to make the most of the view.

Think about these things with regard to your project.

In considering obstacles and advantages, you'll perceive that this image of the tree can be interpreted in two ways. In one sense, you can understand the tree to represent the objective, external situation with regard to the thing you want. In another sense, *you are the tree.* It is your particular assemblage of physical and psychic attributes, helpful and the reverse, that has put you where you are. It is your age, circumstances, horoscope, biorhythms, known and unknown factors of all kinds, which set your schedule for success. So consider both the objective, external factors and the subjective, internal ones.

But when you've weighed it all up, if this is what you really want, don't be discouraged by even the worst apparent chances of success. You need to look at those obstacles — not to dwell upon them — just so you, and your Deep Mind, will know what likely needs to be overcome. *But, when your Deep Mind gets to work on the matter, these obstacles can be overcome — or simply avoided — in ways of which your rational consciousness at present has no idea.*

Your Picture of the Wishing Tree

Make a drawing of the Wishing Tree, like the one

opposite, but, preferably, poster size. Centrally in the roots of the tree, write plainly and concisely the particular good thing you are aiming for as the "fruit" of this practice.

Further up, where the downward-pointing, spiky branches are, write the factors which (after some consideration) you believe to be the chief obstacles which could prevent your gaining this good. Then go a little higher, to the strong, upward-reaching branches, and write there the factors you consider most likely to help you in reaching your objective.

Setting a time by which you want to have achieved this objective is a strong and reasonable way of bringing it within terms of earthly reality. Time is measured by clocks, by heartbeats, by the turning of the Earth and the movements of sun and moon. As soon as you get away from material measurement, you get away from time. In the world of emotion, time goes fast when you are happy; it drags when you are unhappy or bored. If you become engrossed in any occupation, time seems to stand still. The world of the Divine is the world of eternity — of endless dynamic Becoming. So don't be afraid to set a *time* by which you want to have achieved this objective here on Earth. Here you can write a year, or even an exact date, or "My —th birthday", or "—weeks (months, years) from now".

At the top, where the mass of leaves is outlined, place a picture to represent you in possession and enjoyment of the good you want to reach by this practice. This can be a photo if you have a suitable one (for instance, you may have been photographed holding a friend's violin, but your secret wish is to be able really to play; or you may have a vacation picture of yourself sitting on a horse, or at the controls of an airplane, or standing on a high diving board, or whatever, and you want that activity to be a genuine part of your life). Or it can be a magazine clipping, so long as it's something with which you can spontaneously identify: part of a

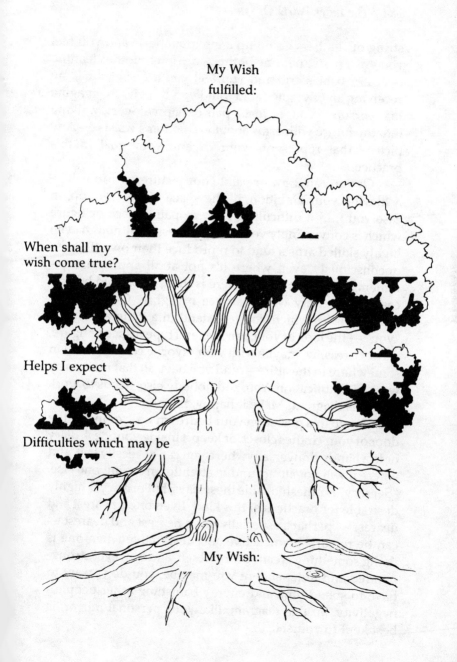

My Wish
fulfilled:

When shall my
wish come true?

Helps I expect

Difficulties which may be

My Wish:

string of climbers going up a mountain face, and you feel you are a particular one of them, a young mother leaning over her babe's crib and you feel you are she, someone receiving an Olympic "gold", and you can vividly imagine that person is you; or just a pair of happy lovers, walking into the future with arms about each other's waists . . . Any picture that represents your dream, your goal in this practice.

Or you can draw or paint your picture, as you will be achieving your ambition, in the space of the tree-top. In case you find it difficult to draw or paint a face or figure which is convincingly your own likeness — although even highly skilled artists tend to reproduce their own likeness unconsciously even where it's not at all appropriate — remember, all that matters here is that you should be able easily to identify with that face or figure. Give it some characteristics which you feel stand in a general way for "you" — the look of your hair, general type of face or figure, way of dressing, maybe with your favorite color painted in somewhere in the attire — and you have all that matters by way of identification. You, and nobody else, needs to work with this diagram! Make it happy, radiant.

Put up this poster on your bedroom wall, or inside the door of your clothes closet, or keep it inside your desk diary or in a handy drawer; anywhere you can get easily to it, and where it will not attract undue attention from anyone else. "Secrecy" is unfashionable these days, but privacy is highly desirable for practices of this kind. Even one's nearest and dearest — perhaps especially one's nearest and dearest — can be remarkably negative and destructive when one is doing something creative for oneself, and however strong-minded and independent you may be, you don't want to have to spend time and energy banishing other people's negativity. So this diagram, like your personal mirror, is best kept to yourself.

Using your "Wishing Tree" with Mirror Power

The Wishing Tree can be a very potent instrument for psychic force, even if you use it by itself; spending, say, twenty minutes daily sitting looking at it, with your Rhythmic Breathing established, and in imagination making your way from the stated objective at the root of the tree, slowly up through the obstacles, slowly up through the helping factors, to the fulfillment of your wish at the top. Only, when you come to the top, take care to think *"This will be"*, not "I wish this might be". But you can make it even more powerful, crisply and mightily effective, if you combine it with a couple of other psychic techniques which entail no difficulty at all.

To begin with, in doing your daily twenty minutes' progress up the Wishing Tree, when you are looking at the picture of the top you can say something like —

My faithful ally, Mirror Friend,

Through you my plans reach joyful end!

Or, if you prefer,

My Mirror Friend, my secret soul,

You help me win my dearest goal!

Whatever you choose, say the same thing every day when you come to the top of the Wishing Tree. And every morning, when you greet your mirror friend with a smile in your personal mirror, say the same words again.

You can repeat the procedure with the mirror several times in the day if you wish, but the procedure with the Wishing Tree picture should be done once a day only.

Nundiales

(If you make that word rhyme with "Gonzalez" you can't be far wrong.)

Should you so desire, there's no reason why you should not go on using this technique of the Wishing Tree, linked with your personal mirror, every day until that particular objective is fulfilled. But it is much more efficient, and it expresses a firmer confidence in the fact that *this will work,* if you do it for just a predetermined number of days and then leave your Deep Mind to take it from there.

But how many days?

You may know about the practice which has long been regarded as one of the special practices of the Roman Church, that of the "novena" as it is nowadays called. That word means simply "a set of nine". Essentially, the practice consists of this: a person who greatly desires some material or spiritual benefit (no matter what) selects nine consecutive days, either at personal convenience, or the nine days leading up to some particular religious festival, or a series of nine days publicly proclaimed for the purpose by the Church or by one of the religious Orders. During that time, the petitioner daily recites certain prescribed prayers, for the "intention" of gaining the desired benefit. This seemingly arbitrary devotion has survived through the centuries because it is extremely powerful; it works.

So ancient is it, in fact, that Christian Rome took it over from Pagan Rome, and Pagan Rome took it from the Etruscans who were acknowledged masters of mystical and psychic lore in the ancient world. In Pagan Rome, much of whose language has descended one way and another into English, this technique was called *Nundiales,* which, if you look at it, refers plainly to *nine days.*

This ages-old insistence on the number nine for the successful working of this technique, gives us some insight into its inner working. The Sphere of the Moon — that is, the mode of consciousness and activity related to the special concerns of the Moon — is known in Qabalistic lore as Yesod, the Ninth Sephirah. Nine is everywhere recognized as a powerful Moon-number; for the Moon presides over all generation and fruitfulness, and, as a traditional Hebrew counting song reminds us, "Nine the months preceding childbirth".

Nine is thus, in all human affairs, the number for the successful gestation and bringing to fruition of any enterprise. So let us see how this ancient and ever-potent technique, which has flourished under, or independently of, the auspices of at least three very different religions (the Etruscan, the Roman and the Christian — nobody knows where it started) can be explicitly re-linked with the lunar source of its power.

Making Use of Moon Symbols

All harvest-bearing trees — fruit trees or nut trees — represent the power of the Moon because of their connotations of fecundity and productiveness. Our Wishing Tree shows forth the lunar influence similarly, since it exists to bring abundance and good gifts into our lives: bringing into material manifestation the abundance of the astral world. Furthermore, the Moon is the "mirror" and in some sense the likeness of the Sun; so our linking of mirror power with the power of the photograph or other likeness is likewise a procedure which comes within the presidency of the Moon. These are in themselves important facts, adding force to our implementation of what we are here doing by the technique of the Nundiales.

We can strengthen this cord of actions and ideas still further, by care taken about the choice of the nine days for its employment. *We can choose nine days which culminate in a Full Moon.*

A calendar which gives the Phases of the Moon makes this easy. Choose a period when you will be able to do your nine days consecutively without interruption. You would not, for instance, go away for a weekend in the middle of the series. (Should you by some unforeseen chance be unable to complete the nine days consecutively, you must in the painstaking manner of the ancient world begin again from the beginning on another occasion.) Find the appropriate day of the Full Moon, and — counting that as "one", count back nine days. The day for which you say "nine" will be the first day of your Nundiales.

(For instance: there was a Full Moon on Friday, May 23, 1986. Counting back through nine days from and including that day, you come to Thursday, May 15. That would be the first day on which to use your Wishing Tree diagram, made out for the specific objective you had in mind at that time; linking the technique with your personal mirror by means of the special greeting and affirmation of success.)

On the final day, that of the Full Moon, simply carry out the same procedure as on the other days, and conclude in full confidence that you have secured the fulfillment of your wish, by whatever means it will be brought to pass on the material level. In the evening of that day, however, it will be a gracious act if you go out of doors when the Full Moon is risen, to give greeting in these or other words, as you may choose:

Lady Moon, Mother of Magick and of Mystery, I salute you on the day of your plenitude. Gently and serenely you watch over your children and illumine their way through the darkness; bounteously you bring them fulfillment of their desires. I affirm in loving confidence that the object of my earnest endeavor will be granted me, and when this shall come to pass, I will behold it, along with the fruits of the earth and the tides of the ocean, as one more sure manifestation of your splendor and your power.

A Mirror for the Nundiales

If the idea of the Nundiales appeals to you, you may wish to make it a frequent feature in your life. In that case, the dedication of a special mirror — not to be used for any other purpose even by you — would be desirable. A wall mirror can be used, or a large hand mirror — preferably round — is particularly to be favored as having the sanction of ancient tradition.

Have ready an adequate piece of soft black material, or a slip-case of the same, in which the mirror can be shielded from the light when not in use.

Naturally, this mirror will be dedicated to the Moon. To this end, charge some water with the planetary power of the Moon, as directed in Chapter 4. If you want to give this dedication something over and above the essentials, take (as may be most convenient to you) a small quantity — say a teaspoonful — of powdered orris root, ginger root, or mugwort (Artemisia) herb, or nine melon seeds or nine jasmine flowers. Boil a cupful of spring water, pour it upon your chosen lunar botanical, let it cool, then strain or filter if necessary. Charge this infusion with the planetary power of the moon.

Wash the surface of your Moon mirror with the charged water or infusion, using your fingers — not a sponge or cloth — and taking care not to let the liquid run into the frame (this for merely practical reasons of not damaging the mirror). Allow it to dry, then place in its black cover until a night of the Full Moon. When the Moon is bright and clear, take off the cover, catch the rays of the Moon in the mirror, and say these or any suitable words you may prefer:

> Lady of watchfulness,
> Lady of dreaming,
> Over the darkened land
> Bright is your beaming!
> As this glass takes your fire,
> With your power fill it:
> Ever my heart's desire
> Be as I will it!

Put the mirror back in its cover, and keep it covered until needed for its purpose.

You should not drink any remaining infusion which has been charged for the dedication. It should be poured upon the earth.

The Other Side of the Conversation

But supposing your Deep Mind has something to say about your plans for the future, or about your program for radiant fitness, more than can be conveyed to you in a simple emotional reaction?

Here, we are once again on common ground with the Formula of the Simulacrum, at the state after the simulacrum has been re-absorbed. In that case, and in this, there is a need to watch developments in the dream life, which is where the Deep Self makes known its own side of any dialog with the rational consciousness.

In considering dreams, naturally, we need to take note of *symbol* and *allegory*, since these, rather than words, form the "language", the means of communication, of the Deep Mind. If you take note, and write down your dreams (even the most seemingly meaningless of them), be asssured your Deep Mind will co-operate; should it have anything special to communicate to you, it will do so. Never mind if (as sometimes happens to even skilled interpreters) you can find no key to the symbolism of one particular dream; if the message it conveys is important to the Deep Mind, it will represent the same meaning in different symbolism on another occasion, and in other symbolism again until it finds a form which you *can* interpret. If you've come across the older psychological idea, that dreams are formulated expressly to disguise or conceal certain ideas, you can be assured this is not the case. The Unconscious, the Subconscious, the Deep Mind — whatever one terms it — wants to be understood, wants to convey its message to us; otherwise, it need not impress our consciousness with a memorable dream at all.

The most important clue to the meaning of a dream is often given by its *emotional tone*. To dream you are in a house you lived in years back (for instance) could mean any number of things, but how did you feel to be there in your dream? — pleased, sad, angry, afraid, nostalgic, adventurous? Did you want everything to be as it was, or did this seem a great chance to change something? Did you feel you were there to try to solve a mystery? Your emotional attitude at once gives a particular significance to the events in the dream, to any objects in it which you felt to be symbolic, and so on. When remembering the dream, take care to identify the emotional feeling of it because that is often the first thing to "evaporate". Also, bear in mind no dream is an isolated thing. Occasionally a fantasy or a memory will come up which you just can't relate to the present (and occasionally, indeed, your Deep Mind can want a brief vacation from relating to the present) but usually your present activities, or your present intentions for the future, will afford a very clear clue to the meaning of some obscure piece of imagery.

But don't lose sleep over your dreams. Your dream life should be taken seriously, but not tragically: it's all a part of your own inner world, and you are in charge.

Your Mirror Friend—Full Length

When you have had some practice with your personal mirror (and maybe with your Moon mirror too), you'll find you can greet and work with your mirror friend in any mirror you happen to see. This can have all kinds of important consequences for you, all of which involves that full length mirror we considered earlier.

If you look in that full length mirror for a final check of your appearance before going out, you can say to yourself — with a smile, of course — "Have a wonderful time!" That adds an extra sparkle to your sense of well-being at once. It also enhances your relationship with that full length mirror.

To do your exercises in front of it certainly is a great help, so long as you keep your sense of direction and don't put a barbell through it. Seriously, though, there are plenty of good exercises you can do without a barbell, and the "tonic" of seeing your muscles responding to your inner commands will do more for you than most pieces of equipment.

With most exercises, just "going through the motions" is of little use unless you are aware of which muscles you are supposed to be developing, or stretching, or whatever. In most cases you will be able to find some way of placing yourself so you can *see* the flex or the stretch as well as feeling it, so your Deep Mind can join in the imaginative play and can say within you "Go on — go on! You can do a little more: here, I'll give you the energy for it, I'll give that dull nerve the consciousness to command a few more fibers to join in!" A little way back, you were told that to enlist the help of your Deep Mind on any project you need to be "specific, dramatic, systematic". The full length mirror helps you make your exercise schedule all of those things.

And meanwhile, tell your Mirror Friend in your personal mirror daily, "You are *strong!*" Or "You are *supple!*" Or *graceful,* or *beautiful* — whatever you are working at.

Radiant Fitness and Radiant Fun

Finally, an important few words on your whole program for radiant fitness. You are undertaking it for the purpose of being able to find more happiness, enjoyment, fun in life! — so don't take any part of it just *too* seriously. If you count the calories in practically every meal you have, you can at any rate afford not to count them two or three times a year on special occasions. If you don't often drink alcohol, chances are — if you've never been an alcoholic — that you won't really like the stuff anyway, so having one glass in front of you to sip will do no damage. (But — caution —you could like a second glass better!) If you only eat health foods, and find yourself presented with a surprise birthday outing to Ye Olde Chinese Junk Restaurant, there will surely be something on the menu which will not kill you outright. So with a lot of other things in life. Radiant fitness is for joy in *living*. Have just that, and prosper!

APPENDIX A

On Fasting

Fasting, after having been regarded for many years as strictly the domain of the religious of many persuasions, and of hunger strikers, has begun in recent years to attract a considerable amount of popular interest, whether simply as a variety in life experience, or as a possibly beneficial addition to dietary procedure. There are different forms of fasting, and the questions of what they can do for you are worth exploring.

The form of fasting which seems at the present time to be the most popular — that of having one completely foodless day regularly every week — is for several reasons not greatly to be recommended. For one thing, it *is* a fashion, and as such is completely arbitrary, not particularly adapted to the needs of any individual; and while there may, for most of us, be little harm in giving a contemporary trend a brief whirl, the fact that "everyone" is doing whatever it is does sometimes prevent the whirlers from recognizing as soon as they should if some particular trend isn't their thing.

As a means of slimming, the weekly foodless day is liable to prove something worse than a failure. Not only will the faster eat more the day after to compensate for it, he or she is likely to eat more all the rest of the week for the same reason. It is, moreover, definitely "out" for anyone with a heart condition, a blood sugar problem, or anemia. Slimming should in any case be done slowly, if only to avoid permanently wrinkling the skin. The best plan is to get on to a sensible no-junk, no-appetizers diet, on the lines indicated earlier in this book, and stay on it for (almost) ever.

Another necessary caution about fasting concerns the question of *motivation*. Because of the history of such matters, fasting has in both Eastern and Western cultures developed a sort of halo of virtue, as being a "good" act — that is, a commendable or ethically desirable act — regardless of any other circumstances. No such ready-made ideas ought to be accepted without thought, but some of them do in fact often maintain a kind of irrational authority in unsorted corners of our minds where they linger undetected. Not only should you examine this; above all it is important you should *never* undertake fasting because of a sense of guilt, or as a form of self-punishment. If you have any intention of making yourself suffer, or of letting yourself suffer, you are evidently going to pay less heed than you should to any signals of distress which your body may put out while you are fasting; and such signals, even for the experienced faster, are important.*

It is notable here that even in the old type of religious establishment where fasting is, or was, customary as a form of penance, it is only permitted under supervision of a competent director. The principle is a sound one.

Fasting is in itself, of course, no more a "virtuous act" than going without sleep would be, or passively suffering toothache. There are only too many factors, which are beyond our control, tending to impair the quality of our life, without our voluntarily adding more. However, if you are a person whose physical health is not likely to be damaged thereby, a fast of predetermined and reasonable length could in fact be of moral worth to you, if you chose to employ it to demonstrate *to yourself* your firm resolution in some serious matter. But, to use fasting in that way, it's evidently necessary that you should not be so inured to it (as for instance by the weekly foodless day regimen) that it requires only a minimal effort on your part.

Why, then, should we fast, and in what manner?

*Whatever your apparent state of health, if you desire to do any regular or serious fasting — even in the ways to be described in this appendix — it's advisable to check first with your doctor.

The Positive Value of Fasting

Above all, fasting purifies the system; or rather, it gives the body a good opportunity to purify itself. It should always be realized that the natural tendency is towards good health and radiant fitness. We can help this natural tendency by supplying the necessary energy and sources of energy (a number of which are dealt with in this book) and also by removing obstacles both external and internal. By fasting, we can give the blood and the digestive system time to throw off accumulated wastes and poisons.

This should not need doing on a weekly basis, unless something is very wrong with our way of life. Indeed, one of the most obvious and reasonable motives for doing it at all is to mark the transition from an unsatisfactory state of affairs to a better one, and this may at least partly account for the widespread interest in fasting at the present time, when so many people are coming to a new realization of the need for a good personal program for living.

Anyone who is giving up alcohol or tobacco, for example, is likely to find a fast of effective length to be an excellent way to mark the transition, not only because it frees the body more rapidly than would otherwise be the case from those lingering toxins which give rise to cravings and "withdrawal symptoms", but also because it gives the psyche temporarily a new focus, an objective and even a problem to cope with which is quite different from the old one. In that case, a fast of from three to seven days (depending upon the general stamina) is a good idea.

If a once-for-all transition to a new way of life is not in question, a periodic purification and renewal of the system by fasting may be desired, in which case an effective annual fast may be the best plan.

Orange Fast and Milk Fast

For an effective three-to-seven-day fast, it is not necessary nor, usually, desirable to abstain from nourishment altogether. To take a form of pure food which is limited in kind but not in quantity, for a period varying according to physique and stamina from three through seven days, is a form of fasting which is often recommended. It should not however be practiced more than once or at most twice in a year, nor should more be needed.

Two good forms of this kind of fasting are the orange fast and the milk fast. Both are excellent purifiers. Each one gives you some essential nutrients and deprives you, for the time you are on the fast, of others. That is one reason why, for even the healthiest and fittest person, these — or, indeed, any — fasts should not be prolonged for more than seven days.

Conditions for Fasting

There are some arrangements you should make for your fast.

You should choose a time of warm, bright weather for it. During a fast, your energy is precious and should not need to be expended unduly in replenishing lost body heat. Emotional tone, too, may be lowered during fasting, and sunshine and blue skies help banish depression.

You need to have adequate supplies of your fasting food available, so you can consume as much of it as you want whenever you want. You are likely to feel to some extent afflicted by the monotony of your fasting diet and the lack of a "square meal", but there should be no rationing of the chosen sustenance.

You should also drink plain water when you feel like it, although during this fast there is no need to keep strictly to your six glasses a day.

It is best to be on vacation while fasting because of several of the considerations mentioned above, and also because, for the duration of your liquid diet, the frequency of visits to the bathroom will inevitably be much increased. This, of course, is a good sign of the entire bodily purification which is going on.

Your fast is not a good time for violent activity whether physical or intellectual. It is however an excellent time gently to step up your psychic awareness. If you already meditate, don't break that practice: if you have not taken it up before, this might be a good time to do so. Too, psychic powers such as telepathy or psychometry may come to your attention at this time.

Above all, stay cheerful! Enjoy extra music, or reading, or any non-strenuous pleasure which appeals to you. If possible, avoid anyone who is likely to make a point of trying to talk you out of your resolved plan of action; otherwise; the best treatment for such is during your fast to take extra care with your dress and grooming, and to appear with special glow and sparkle. You can in fact do that very genuinely, and feel all the better for it: reminding yourself—sharing it with your Deep Mind—that you are entering into a new phase of truly good living, of radiant fitness, to which your fast is only the doorway.

APPENDIX B
The Tropical Banana Breakfast

You may now and then have heard it said that a banana for breakfast is good for the figure. If so, you probably did nothing about it. The simple fact, thus stated, is not very impressive: it gives you no idea of how the banana should be eaten so as to give its special benefit, nor, indeed, exactly what you can expect from it.

I have called the vital recipe Tropical because of its associations, as well as for the tropical ingredients which compose it. Besides — imagine! If you were suddenly transported to an ideal beach, your dream Malibu, how would you want to look?

That's a nice little picture to keep illuminated in a corner of your mind, a standard to work to in your progress to Radiant Fitness.

Like some other good diet meals (which are not all so enjoyable), this breakfast is something of a "magical mystery": the reasons why its combination of good things should be so effective are not altogether obvious. But it has worked excellently for a number of people, and deserves to be better known. First, therefore, I will tell of the Breakfast itself and the way I came to know of it; then we can look at what it gives you.

That day, I was having fun looking at the new season's most sumptuous dress fabrics in Harrods, London, and coordinating them in imagination with the lately announced styles. A number of women and men, similarly occupied for personal or professional reasons, were strolling about the spacious department in which the lovely merchandise was displayed.

Absorbed in building my inner pictures, I paid little attention to the passing snatches of conversation in several languages; I appreciated them simply as part of an ambience which was at the same time esthetic and intelligent, urbane and sensuous. Then, in one of those random silences which inevitably focus the attention, a woman's voice, soft toned but vibrant with interest and curiosity, was raised in frank question:

"But how do you keep such a marvelous figure?"

The head of every man or woman within hearing jerked as if on a string for a view of the person thus addressed. My ears, too, were alert for her reply; especially because, having expected to see a fashionable "skinny", I now identified the questioned one as a young woman with a figure truly superb. She had a tan which the most southerly British shores never engendered, and her light, bright wraparound dress heightened the illusion that she had just left a tropical beach. She had the look, too, of a frequent swimmer: there had to be good exercise as well as dieting know-how to account for her perfect and balanced development. A face whose planes radiated character was poised upon a strong, rounded neck; a trim waist separated the splendid curves of bust and hip, while long muscles gave firmness and animation to her graceful limbs. With a little laugh, she replied:

"It's simple. Every morning I cut up a banana and put it in the blender with a spoonful of honey and a spoonful, or a little more, of lemon juice. If you do this and eat it before anything else, you can eat what you like for the rest of the day."

Those are her exact words. They raise several questions, admittedly. In eating "what you like", presumably you allow the effects of this breakfast to influence the kinds and quantities of food you feel inclined to. As with the grapefruit juice (see page 139), the lemon juice, if you don't altogether overwhelm it with honey has a tendency to free the palate from a craving for sweet things. Honey, it may be noted, is never the chosen food of sucrose "addicts"; in fact, far from being a mere substitute for sugar, honey contains fructose and has the great advantage of being absorbed into the system only slowly. Hence the "staying power" of the Breakfast.

The quantities of honey and lemon juice suggested are inexact, but they have to be, since the size and ripeness of bananas are quite variable. With regard to bananas, a few things remain to be said.

An unripe banana is mainly starch. In fact, if you are *not* keen to lose weight and you want to plan a "tropical" meal, unripe banana cut into strips and cooked makes a delicious, authentic and healthful vegetable to accompany meats, sweet-and-sour dishes, kebabs and mixed grills. As a banana ripens, the starch turns to sugar — fructose again, naturally — and it becomes proportionately better for "diet" meals. However, any banana which is in the yellow-skinned condition and is easily peeled, is likely to be suitable for the Breakfast recipe.

If you don't live in banana growing country, your best plan if you can manage it is to buy the fruit for your Tropical Banana Breakfasts every two or three days. That way, you can always have a banana which is ripe, but never too ripe to be attractive. Supposing however you are one of the many people who can only do their grocery shopping once a week?

No harm! There seems to be a widespread belief around, that you can't put bananas in the refrigerator or they will be spoiled: but this is not the case. Certainly the skin begins to darken after a few days, and will become quite black; but the fruit inside will remain white and sweet. Naturally there is a limit to this, and the length of time the bananas will keep depends upon such variables as their degree of ripeness, the room temperature before refrigerating them, and the setting of the refrigerator. But in any particular case it is true that bananas keep fresh, eatable and delicious for considerably longer than they would have done if not refrigerated.

If you don't have a mechanical blender, no problem! If you have teeth, you have a blender; and to many people, the appearance of a small bowl of sliced banana with honey and lemon juice poured over it, is far more attractive than the mixture would be if pulped.

Finally, for a luxurious-tasting tropical change, you might sometimes like to use lime juice instead of lemon.

When you have lost enough weight, you may still want to enjoy your Tropical Banana Breakfast without having it every day. You might for instance enjoy it two or three times in a week: your breakfast on some of the other days could be home-made granola (page 137), on other days cottage cheese topped with raw or cooked fruit. All are healthful, unfattening, and energizing meals.

Good mornings!

APPENDIX C
A Calm Look at AIDS

It often happens that a disease previously unknown, or one which suddenly flares to epidemic proportions, will cause fear and distress far beyond the actual suffering it inflicts, because the idea of it begins to prey upon people's imagination and on their nerves.

Our civilization has always had some particular "bogey". For a long time, through the Middle Ages, the dreaded demon was leprosy, for which the effects of malnutrition were often mistaken. Then it was bubonic plague; then syphilis; then smallpox; then tuberculosis; then cancer. Cancer has not yet been vanquished by medical science, although great advances have been made; but now, in this penultimate decade of the century, its place in the forefront of public apprehension — at any rate in the United States — has been taken by a new disease, *Acquired Immune Deficiency Syndrome*, generally known as AIDS.

All the diseases just named have been, and are, serious killers. The point being made here is that in every case the spread of the disease — and of other diseases, inevitably — was facilitated by the general feeling of fatalism concerning them, and an irrational aura of real superstition, which tended to overshadow the public consciousness. In centuries with less medical understanding than ours, this was excusable; now it is a strangely retrograde attitude.

This irrational fear of a disease — whatever disease — has certain recurring characteristics, some of which are inapplicable here. But we can note that one of the features recurring in history is a tendency to blame a mysterious outbreak of sickness on to some section of people who are unpopular, not understood, often people of different religious or political views. (One of the most curious examples of this is the fable, frequently repeated by historians, attributing the great 15th-16th century outbreak of syphilis in Europe to the Native American captives taken there by Columbus: although those captives were observed to be singularly healthy people, and — more remarkably — although the classic marks of hereditary syphilis were present in at least one famous European family, before Columbus ever made his first voyage. The ubiquitous Oriental-Venetian slave trade was much more likely involved in that matter.)

These things being so, and if for no other reason, the frequently-heard attribution of the origin of AIDS to the male homosexual community is to be regarded with extreme reserve. In a sense, its origin doesn't matter very much now. But it is disastrous that some people imagine, as they seem to, that AIDS is limited to homophiles or that it is a special "divine judgment" upon them. On the medical evidence, if AIDS had a sexual origin at all (and it certainly is not a venereal disease in the limited sense) its development could well have been associated with practices of oral sex which are general, and normal, among lovers of every sort.

Incidentally, the spread of AIDS has been publicly suggested to have another origin. On *that* theory, it would be an act of biological warfare on the part of — guess who?

Let us get to the facts. There is not at the time of writing any known cure for AIDS, and (also at the time of writing) research on this seems to be seriously hampered by a unique lack of funds for the purpose. Those circumstances, we can hope, are both open to rapid change. *Meantime, we can all help the situation — and help it materially — by considering on the one hand how to check the spread of the disease (which includes avoiding catching it ourselves) and on the other hand how to dispel the cloud of misconception, irrational fear and down-*

right superstition which is paralyzing responsible decisions; and which, incidentally, also forms a real breeding-ground of worry and depression to foment every malady that exists.

To begin this positive program, we must take a clear look at the nature of AIDS so far as this is at present known. More about it may become known at any time, and we should possess ourselves of any new facts: making sure they are facts. Rumor and emotionalism should be avoided like a plague — which is just what they are.

AIDS — Acquired Immune Deficiency Syndrome —is a sickness caused by a virus, as influenza and the common cold are also. Some forms of influenza are killers: AIDS is a killer in two ways. A person who contracts this malady is likely in the long run to die of it, unless a cure is discovered before that time; but it has its periods of remission, and the sufferer's fighting chances are at any rate improved by avoidance of depression and fatalism. Also, however, as its name indicates, the virus has a peculiar property of attacking the body's natural defense systems, so as to make the sufferer dangerously vulnerable to even the simplest further infection he or she might contract meanwhile. On the evidence it looks as if such a person might be as defenseless before a common cold, for instance, as were the Martians in H.G. Wells' *War of the Worlds*. But it is to be noted that the words, *Acquired Immune Deficiency Syndrome*, cautiously avoid being absolute. To be deficient in any quality is not necessarily to be totally without it.

Furthermore, AIDS does not appear to be quite as easily transmissible as some forms of virus malady. If your lover gets the 'flu, generally speaking you can be fairly sure to get the 'flu also; but it has been known for one member of a couple to have AIDS, and the other to be free from it. And yet there are some people who have developed AIDS without their source of infection being evident.

It is known that the lymphatic system of the body is involved in the disease (a persistent thirst and a dry cough are among its symptoms), and the saliva is indicated as a likely carrier of the virus. Following this line of thought, a common-sense first line of defence would be to avoid *all* general kissing, no matter how innocently motivated. As a noted psychologist pointed out in a recently televised debate on AIDS, "We are dealing with *a virus*, not with a question of morals."

If this line of thinking on AIDS should become established, it might become general and reasonable practice, as in the Middle Ages, for each person when eating out to carry his or her own cup and flatware, or for "once-only" items to be provided at restaurants. In emergency circumstances this would not be considered eccentric, and would in fact prevent many infections besides the one we are discussing.

It is on the mental and emotional side, however, that our defences can here and now be of the greatest importance and value.

Your objective is not only to avoid AIDS, but also to preserve your health unimpaired by any sickness. Already, with regard to bacterial diseases at least, it is a proven fact that to reduce stress and anxiety is to increase very considerably the body's resistance to infection. In respect to the viruses we have no such clear picture as yet, but the physical results of relaxation — better oxygenated blood, less fatigue, more energy — must in all circumstances count in a person's favor.

Good diet, besides conferring its intrinsic benefits, helps further by promoting stronger nerves and better relaxation. The program outlined in this book, with as much fresh air and exercise as your personal schedule allows, is the best possible safeguard against AIDS or any other infection.

But what about your sex life?

Be prudent, but don't make a nightmare of your own life or of anyone else's.

AIDS is not a venereal disease. Nor is it a "judgment of God" on anyone. It is simply and solely a virus: one which is not well understood as yet.

Don't be rash or promiscuous. To be promiscuous, or to have a lover who is so, is to enlarge immensely your number of contacts, or contacts one or two steps removed, any one of whom may be a carrier of some infection or other.

At the same time *don't worry* about a possibility of infection from your lover. This is important. If you can't stop worrying, you'd best stop having sex. Nobody can enjoy making love to a tense, preoccupied woman or man, and sex without pleasure is a pernicious cause of depression in anyone's life. If on the other hand you feel your love is important to go on with, then pull yourself together and turn your mind from those dark imaginings. Relax. Live for every moment of your lovemaking. Tension and anxiety are altogether negative, and can do nothing good for you.

Take stock of the situation therefore, and make sober and positive decisions as to your best course of action. Build yourself up, body and soul, with good food, exercise, sleep, meditation, fresh air and contact with the world of nature; with happiness and with love. Fortify yourself too with the Magick that is in all these things, and radiate your well-being to the world.

Be strong, be fit — and live!

STAY IN TOUCH

On the following pages you will find listed, with their current prices, some of the books and tapes now available on related subjects. Your book dealer stocks most of these, and will stock new titles in the Llewellyn series as they become available. We urge your patronage.

However, to obtain our full catalog, to keep informed of new titles as they are released and to benefit from informative articles and helpful news, you are invited to write for our bi-monthly news magazine/catalog. A sample copy is free, and it will continue coming to you at no cost as long as you are an active mail customer. Or you may keep it coming for a full year with a donation of just $2.00 in U.S.A. ($7.00 for Canada & Mexico, $10.00 overseas, first class mail). Many bookstores also have *The Llewellyn New Times* available to their customers. Ask for it.

Stay in touch! In *The Llewellyn New Times'* pages you will find news and reviews of new books, tapes and services, announcements of meetings and seminars, articles helpful to our readers, news of authors, advertising of products and services, special money-making opportunities, and much more.

The Llewellyn New Times
P.O. Box 64383-Dept. 165, St. Paul, MN 55164-0383, U.S.A.

• • •

TO ORDER BOOKS AND TAPES

If your book dealer does not have the books and tapes described on the following pages readily available, you may order them direct from the publisher by sending full price in U.S. funds, plus $1.00 for handling and 50¢ each book or item for postage within the United States; outside USA surface mail add $1.00 extra per item. Outside USA air mail add $7.00 per item.

FOR GROUP STUDY AND PURCHASE

Because there is a great deal of interest in group discussion and study of the subject matter of this book, we feel that we should encourage the adoption and use of this particular book by such groups by offering a special "quantity" price to group leaders or "agents".

Our Special Quality Price for a minimum order of five copies of THE INNER WORLD OF FITNESS is $23.85 Cash-With-Order. This price includes postage and handling within the United States. Minnesota residents must add 6% sales tax. For additional quantities, please order in multiples of five. For Canadian and foreign orders, add postage and handling charges as above. Credit Card (VISA, MasterCard, American Express, Diners' Club) Orders are accepted. Charge Card Orders only may be phoned free ($15.00 minimum order) within the U.S.A. by dialing 1-800-THE MOON (in Canada call: 1-800-FOR-SELF). Customer Service calls dial 1-612-291-1970 and ask for "Kae". Mail Orders to:

LLEWELLYN PUBLICATIONS
P.O. Box 64383-Dept. 165 / St. Paul, MN 55164-0383, U.S.A.

**THE LLEWELLYN PRACTICAL GUIDE
TO ASTRAL PROJECTION.**
by Melita Denning & Osborne Phillips
Yes, your consciousness can be sent forth, out-of-the-body, with full awareness and return with full memory. You can travel through time and space, converse with non-physical entities, obtain knowledge by non-material means, and experience higher dimensions.

> **Is there life-after-death? Are we forever shackled by Time & Space? The ability to go forth by means of the Astral Body, or Body of Light, gives the personal assurance of consciousness (and life) beyond the limitations of the physical body.**

The reader is led through the essential stages for the inner growth and development that will culminate in fully conscious projection and return. Not only are the requisite practices set forth in step-by-step procedures, augmented with photographs and puts-you-in-the-picture" visualization aids, but the vital reasons for undertaking them are clearly explained. Beyond this, the great benefits from the various practices themselves are demonstrated in renewed physical and emotional health, mental discipline, spiritual attainment, and the development of extra faculties".

Guidance is also given to the Astral World itself: what to expect, what can be done—including the ecstatic experience of Astral Sex.

0-87542-181-4, 239 pages, 5¼ x 8, softcover   **$7.95**

**THE LLEWELLYN PRACTICAL GUIDE
TO CREATIVE VISUALIZATION**
by Melita Denning & Osborne Phillips
All things you will ever want must have their start in your mind. The average person uses very little of the full creative power that is his, potentially. It's like the power locked in the atom—it's all there, but you have to learn to release it and apply it constructively.

> **If you can see it in your Mind's Eye, you will have it! It's true: you can have whatever you want—but there are "laws" to Mental Creation that must be followed. The power of the mind is not limited to, nor limited by, the Material World—Creative Visualization enables Man to reach beyond, into the Invisible World of Astral and Spiritual Forces.**

Some people apply this innate power without actually knowing what they are doing, and achieve great success and happiness; most people, however, use this same power, again unknowingly, INCORRECTLY, and experience bad luck, failure, or at best unfulfilled life.
This book changes that. Through an easy series of step-by-step, progressive exercises, your mind is applied to bring desire into realization! You can easily develop this completely natural power, and correctly apply it, for your immediate and practical benefit. Illustrated with unique, "puts-you-into-the-picture" visualization aids.

0-87542-183-0, 255 pages, 5¼ x 8, softcover.   **$7.95**

THE ART OF SPIRITUAL HEALING
by Keith Sherwood

Each of you has the potential to be a healer; to heal yourself and to become a channel for healing others. Healing energy is always flowing through you. Learn how to recognize and tap this incredible energy source. Rid yourself of negativity and become a channel for positive healing.

Special techniques make this book a "breakthrough" to healing power, but you are also given a concise, easy-to-follow regimen of good health to follow in order to maintain a superior state of being.

0-87542-720-0, softcover, illustrated. **$7.95**

THE WOMEN'S SPIRITUALITY BOOK
by Diane Stein

Diane Stein's forthcoming release (December 1986) of THE WOMEN'S SPIRITUALITY BOOK, is a work of insight and a much needed addition to women's magic and ritual. Beginning with "Creation and Creation Goddesses" she enthusiastically informs the reader of the essence of women-centered Wicca, using myths and legends drawn from a variety of world sources to bring her work to life.

The second half of the book is a valuable introduction to visualization, healing, chakras, crystal and gemstone magick. Subsequent chapters cover "transformational tarot" and Kwan Yin.

Diane Stein's WOMEN'S SPIRITUALITY BOOK is a tool for self-discovery and initiation into the Higher Self: a joyous reunion with the Goddess.

0-87542-761-8, 300 pages, 5¼ x 8, softcover. **$9.95**

PRACTICAL COLOR MAGICK by Raymond Buckland

The world is a rainbow of color, a symphony of vibration. We have left the Newtonian idea of the world as being made of large mechanical units, and now know it as a strange chaos of vibrations ordered by our senses, but, our senses are limited and designed by Nature to give us access to only those vibratory emanations we need for survival.

But, we live far from the natural world now. And the colors which filled our habitats when we were natural creatures have given way to grey and black and synthetic colors of limited wave lengths determined not by our physiological needs but by economic constraints.

Raymond Buckland, author of the world-famous PRACTICAL CANDLE BURNING RITUALS has produced a fascinating and useful new book, PRACTICAL COLOR MAGICK which shows you how to reintroduce color into your life to benefit your physical, mental and spiritual well-being!

PRACTICAL COLOR MAGICK will teach all the powers of light and more! You'll learn new forms of expression of your inner-most self, new ways of relating to others with the secret languages of light and color.

0-87542-047-8, 136 pages, softcover, illustrated **$5.95**